# Hematopoietic Stem Cell Transplantation for Immunodeficiency, Part II

*Guest Editor*

CHAIM M. ROIFMAN, MD, FRCPC, FCACB

# IMMUNOLOGY AND ALLERGY CLINICS OF NORTH AMERICA

www.immunology.theclinics.com

*Consulting Editor*
RAFEUL ALAM, MD, PhD

May 2010 • Volume 30 • Number 2

SAUNDERS an imprint of ELSEVIER, Inc.

**W.B. SAUNDERS COMPANY**

*A Division of Elsevier Inc.*

1600 John F. Kennedy Blvd., • Suite 1800 • Philadelphia, PA 19103-2899.

http://www.theclinics.com

**IMMUNOLOGY AND ALLERGY CLINICS OF NORTH AMERICA Volume 30, Number 2**
**May 2010 ISSN 0889–8561, ISBN-13: 978-1-4377-1829-4**

Editor: Patrick Manley

*Immunology and Allergy Clinics of North America* (ISSN 0889–8561) is published quarterly by Elsevier Inc., 360 Park Avenue South, New York, NY 10010-1710. Months of issue are February, May, August, and November. Periodicals postage paid at New York, NY and additional mailing offices. Subscription prices are $254.00 per year for US individuals, $373.00 per year for US institutions, $123.00 per year for US students and residents, $312.00 per year for Canadian individuals, $178.00 per year for Canadian students, $463.00 per year for Canadian institutions, $354.00 per year for international individuals, $463.00 per year for international institutions, $178.00 per year for international students. To receive student/resident rate, orders must be accompanied by name of affiliated institution, date of term, and the *signature* of program/residency coordinator on institution letterhead. Orders will be billed at individual rate until proof of status is received. Foreign air speed delivery is included in all *Clinics* subscription prices. All prices are subject to change without notice. **POSTMASTER**: Send address changes to *Immunology and Allergy Clinics of North America,* Elsevier Health Sciences Division, Subscription Customer Service, 3251 Riverport Lane, Maryland Heights, MO 63043. **Customer Service: 1-800-654-2452 (U.S. and Canada); 314-447-8871 (outside U.S. and Canada). Fax: 314-447-8029. E-mail: journalscustomerservice-usa@elsevier.com (for print support); journalsonlinesupport-usa@elsevier.com (for online support).**

*Reprints.* For copies of 100 or more, of articles in this publication, please contact the Commercial Reprints Department, Elsevier Inc., 360 Park Avenue South, New York, New York 10010-1710. Tel. (212) 633-3812, Fax: (212) 462-1935, e-mail: reprints@elsevier.com.

*Immunology and Allergy Clinics of North America is covered in MEDLINE/PubMed (Index Medicus), Current Contents/Life Sciences, Science Citation Index, ISI/BIOMED, Chemical Abstracts, and EMBASE/Excerpta Medica.*

Printed and bound by CPI Group (UK) Ltd, Croydon, CR0 4YY

Transferred to Digital Print 2011

# Contributors

## CONSULTING EDITOR

**RAFEUL ALAM, MD, PhD**
Veda and Chauncey Ritter Chair in Immunology, Professor, and Director, Division
of Immunology and Allergy, National Jewish Health; and University of Colorado
Health Sciences Center, Denver, Colorado

## GUEST EDITOR

**CHAIM M. ROIFMAN, MD, FRCPC, FCACB**
Donald and Audrey Campbell Chair of Immunology; Head, Division of Immunology
& Allergy, The Canadian Centre for Primary Immunodeficiency, The Jeffrey Modell
Research Laboratory for the Diagnosis of Primary Immunodeficiency, The Hospital
for Sick Children, University of Toronto, Toronto, Ontario, Canada

## AUTHORS

**ALESSANDRO AIUTI, MD, PhD**
Associate Professor of Pediatrics, San Raffaele Telethon Institute for Gene Therapy
(HSR-TIGET); Pediatric Immunohematology and Bone Marrow Transplantation Unit,
San Raffaele Scientific Institute, Milan; Department of Pediatrics, Children's Hospital
Bambino Gesù, University of Rome Tor Vergata, Rome, Italy

**BARBARA CAPPELLI, MD**
San Raffaele Telethon Institute for Gene Therapy (HSR-TIGET); Pediatric
Immunohematology and Bone Marrow Transplantation Unit, San Raffaele Scientific
Institute, Milan, Italy

**M. CAVAZANNA-CALVO, MD, PhD**
Developpement normal et pathologique du systeme immunitaire, Inserm U 768;
Paris-Descartes University; Department of Biotherapy, Hopital Necker-Enfants Malades,
Assistance Publique-Hôpitaux de Paris (AP-HP), Université René Descartes; INSERM,
Centre d'Investigation Clinique intégré en Biothérapies, Groupe Hospitalier Universitaire
Ouest, AP-HP, Paris, France

**AGNIESZKA CZECHOWICZ, BS**
MD/PhD Student, Institute of Stem Cell Biology and Regenerative Medicine, Stanford
University School of Medicine, Stanford, California

**M. TERESA DE LA MORENA, MD**
Associate Professor of Pediatrics and Internal Medicine, Division of Allergy and
Immunology, University of Texas Southwestern Medical Center in Dallas, Dallas, Texas

**ALAIN FISCHER, MD, PhD**
University Paris Descartes, Necker Medical School; Institut National de la Santé et de la Recherche Médicale; Unité d'Immuno-Hématologie Pédiatrique, Necker Hospital, Assistance Publique-Hôpitaux de Paris, Paris, France

**H. BOBBY GASPAR, MRCP(UK), PhD, MRCPCH**
Centre for Immunodeficiency, Molecular Immunology Unit, UCL Institute of Child Health, London, United Kingdom

**S. HACEIN-BEY-ABINA, PharmD, PhD**
Developpement normal et pathologique du systeme immunitaire, Inserm U 768; Paris-Descartes University; Department of Biotherapy, Hopital Necker-Enfants Malades, Assistance Publique-Hôpitaux de Paris (AP-HP), Université René Descartes; INSERM, Centre d'Investigation Clinique intégré en Biothérapies, Groupe Hospitalier Universitaire Ouest, AP-HP, Paris, France

**LUIGI D. NOTARANGELO, MD**
Harvard Medical School; Division of Immunology and The Manton Center for Orphan Disease Research, Children's Hospital Boston, Karp Family Research Laboratories, Boston, Massachusetts

**SUNG-YUN PAI, MD**
Division of Hematology-Oncology, Children's Hospital Boston, Karp Family Research Laboratories; Department of Pediatric Oncology, Dana-Farber Cancer Institute; Harvard Medical School, Boston, Massachusetts

**CAPUCINE PICARD, MD, PhD**
Study Center of Primary Immunodeficiencies, Necker Hospital, Assistance Publique-Hôpitaux de Paris; Laboratory of Human Genetics of Infectious Diseases, Institut National de la Santé et de la Recherche Médicale; University Paris Descartes, Necker Medical School, Paris, France

**CHAIM M. ROIFMAN, MD, FRCPC, FCACB**
Donald and Audrey Campbell Chair of Immunology; Head, Division of Immunology & Allergy, The Canadian Centre for Primary Immunodeficiency, The Jeffrey Modell Research Laboratory for the Diagnosis of Primary Immunodeficiency, The Hospital for Sick Children, University of Toronto, Toronto, Ontario, Canada

**REINHARD A. SEGER, MD**
Division of Immunology/Hematology/BMT, University Children's Hospital, Zürich, Switzerland

**IRVING L. WEISSMAN, MD**
Director, Institute of Stem Cell Biology and Regenerative Medicine, Stanford University School of Medicine, Stanford, California

# Contents

Replacement of disease-causing stem cells with healthy ones has been achieved clinically via hematopoietic cell transplantation (HCT) for the last 40 years, as a treatment modality for a variety of cancers and immunodeficiencies with moderate, but increasing, success. This procedure has traditionally included transplantation of mixed hematopoietic populations that include hematopoietic stem cells (HSC) and other cells, such as T cells. This article explores and delineates the potential expansion of this technique to treat a variety of inherited diseases of immune function, the current barriers in HCT and pure HSC transplantation, and the up-and-coming strategies to combat these obstacles.

Major histocompatibility complex (MHC) class II expression deficiency is a rare condition with autosomal recessive transmission. The defect of MHC class II leads to combined immunodeficiency with defective CD4$^+$ T-cell development and a lack of T helper cell–dependent antibody production by B cells. The clinical course of disease is characterized by the recurrence of bacterial, viral, fungal, and protozoan infections. The optimal symptomatic care that is available involves the prophylactic use of antibiotics and the administration of immunoglobulin with adequate nutritional support. Hematopoietic stem cell transplantation is the only known treatment available to cure MHC class II expression deficiency.

The Wiskott-Aldrich syndrome (WAS) is an X-linked disorder characterized by a triad of diagnostic clinical elements: immunodeficiency, eczema, and hemorrhage caused by thrombocytopenia with small-sized platelets. Hematopoietic cell transplantation (HCT) can cure WAS, and is most often performed using myeloablative conditioning regimens. Our growing

understanding of the biology of WASp has revealed cell-type specific functions that impact immune and hematopoietic outcome after HCT. Short-
and long-term toxicities associated with HCT remain the main obstacle
to safe and effective cure for every patient with WAS. Optimal management strategies for patients with milder forms of the disease (including
X-linked thrombocytopenia) remain to be defined.

Chronic granulomatous disease (CGD) is a primary immunodeficiency disease that is caused by the lack of 1 of 5 subunits of the superoxide-producing nicotinamide adenine dinucleotide phosphate oxidase of
neutrophils, macrophages, and eosinophils. Allogeneic hematopoietic
stem cell transplantation (HSCT) is currently the only curative treatment
for CGD and can be offered to selected patients. Improved outcome
with supportive care and high clinical variability in the disease course,
however, make selection of eligible patients for HSCT difficult. This article
addresses recent progress in HSCT for CGD, delineates present limitations, and points to future developments.

Typical cases of severe combined immunodeficiency present at infancy
(most frequently at 6 months of age) with repeated opportunistic infections; failure to thrive; and scarcity of lymphoid tissues, including undetectable lymph nodes and a small dysplastic thymus. Patients with profound
T-cell dysfunction (PTD)/combined immunodeficiency (CID) have moderate to large numbers of circulating autologous lymphocytes with variable
residual function. These cells may interfere with proper engraftment and
may complicate the procedure of HSCT, hence the need for conditioning.
There is no immediate explanation for the excellent outcome of hematopoietic stem cell transplantation (HSCT) for PTD/CID. Historically, protocols for mismatched related donor HSCT did not include conditioning
regimens, which could jeopardize engraftment. Careful studies on the
role of conditioning, especially myeloablative conditioning, should be conducted in the future. It is possible that in some genotypes, related identical
donor can be accepted by the recipient with little or no conditioning. Until
such studies become instructive, the protocols in current use seem to provide excellent, although not perfect, outcome in patients with PTD/CID.

Adenosine deaminase (ADA)-deficient severe combined immunodeficiency (SCID) comprises approximately 10% to 15% of all cases of
SCID. The clinical effects of ADA deficiency are manifest most dramatically
in the immune system, where it leads to severe lymphopenia. Although hematopoietic stem cell transplantation remains the mainstay of treatment

for ADA-deficient SCID, 2 other treatment options are available, namely enzyme replacement therapy with PEG-ADA and autologous hematopoietic stem cell gene therapy. In this article the author reviews the available data on treatment by these different options, and offers an overview on when each of the different treatment options should be used.

The concept of gene therapy emerged as a way of correcting monogenic inherited diseases by introducing a normal copy of the mutated gene into at least some of the patients' cells. Although this concept has turned out to be quite complicated to implement, it is in the field of primary immunodeficiencies (PIDs) that proof of feasibility has been undoubtedly achieved. There is now a strong rationale in support of gene therapy for at least some PIDs, as discussed in this article.

In the last decade, gene therapy for adenosine deaminase deficiency has been developed as a successful alternative strategy to allogeneic bone marrow transplant and enzyme replacement therapy. Infusion of autologous hematopoietic stem cells, corrected ex vivo by retroviral vectors and combined to low-intensity conditioning regimen, has resulted in immunologic improvement, metabolic correction, and long-term clinical benefits. These findings have opened the way to applications of gene therapy in other primary immune deficiencies using novel vector technology.

A complete list of definite, as well as possible, indications for hemopoietic stem cell transplantation in primary immunodeficiency is provided. Included are: severe combined immunodeficiency, profound T cell defects, autoimmune and autoinflammatory syndromes, innate immune defects, hemophagocytic disorders, and other conditions. Some causes and limitations are included.

## FORTHCOMING ISSUES

### August 2010
**Atopic Dermatitis**
Mark Boguniewicz, MD, *Guest Editor*

### November 2010
**Infectious Diseases and Asthma**
Gary Hellermann, MD, and
Shyam Mohapatra, MD,
*Guest Editors*

### February 2011
**Stress and Immune-Based Diseases**
Gailen D. Marshall, MD,
*Guest Editor*

## RECENT ISSUES

### February 2010
**Hematopoietic Stem Cell Transplantation
for Immunodeficiency, Part I**
Chaim M. Roifman, MD, FRCPC, FCACB,
*Guest Editor*

### November 2009
**Chronic Rhinosinusitis**
Wystke J. Fokkens, MD, *Guest Editor*

### August 2009
**Drug Hypersensitivity**
Werner J. Pichler, MD, *Guest Editor*

---

**RELATED INTEREST**

*Pediatric Clinics of North America* (Volume 57, Issue 1, Pages 1–352, February 2010)
**Hematopoietic Stem Cell Transplantation**
Max J. Coppes, MD, PhD, MBA, Terry J. Fry, MD, and Crystal L. Mackall, MD,
*Guest Editors*

---

## THE CLINICS ARE NOW AVAILABLE ONLINE!

Access your subscription at:
**www.theclinics.com**

# Foreword

# Hematopoietic Stem Cell Transplantation for Primary Immunodeficiency Disorders, Part II

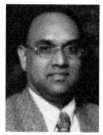

Rafeul Alam, MD, PhD
*Consulting Editor*

A quick review of the literature indicates that among all the areas of medical sciences, immunodeficiency seems to have benefited the most from the advances in the gene sequencing technology and from the human genome project. The speed of the progress is astounding. Within the first 3 months of 2010, I counted more than 25 publications in PubMed directly related to new mutations in immunodeficiency disorders. This accelerated progress is likely due to the fact that many immunodeficiency disorders result from a single gene defect. This is unlike complex diseases, such as asthma or type 2 diabetes mellitus, which are likely polygenic. The single gene mutation in immunodeficiency disorders makes them ideal candidates for gene therapy. The major hurdle to gene therapy has been the selection of an appropriate vector. Retroviral and adenoviral vectors have their advantages and disadvantages. Viral insertion-related proto-oncogene activation and its adverse consequences as well as vector silencing through methylation remain major problems.[1–3] Until these problems are solved, hematopoietic stem cell transplantation remains a valuable

Supported by NIH grants RO1 AI059719 and AI68088, PPG HL 36577 and N01 HHSN272200700048C.

Immunol Allergy Clin N Am 30 (2010) ix–x
doi:10.1016/j.iac.2010.03.005
0889-8561/10/$ – see front matter
immunology.theclinics.com

therapeutic option. This is Part II of hematopoietic stem cell transplantation. Under the editorship of Dr Roifman, this issue covers topics related to hematopoietic stem cell transplantation in profound T-cell deficiency and combined immunodeficiency.

Rafeul Alam, MD, PhD
Division of Allergy & Immunology
National Jewish Health & University of Colorado
Denver Health Sciences Center
1400 Jackson Street, Denver, CO 80206, USA

E-mail address:
alamr@njc.org

## REFERENCES

1. Hacein-Bey-Abina S, Von Kalle C, Schmidt M, et al. LMO2-associated clonal T cell proliferation in two patients after gene therapy for SCID-X1. Science 2003;302: 415–9.
2. Hacein-Bey-Abina S, Garrigue A, Wang GP, et al. Insertional oncogenesis in 4 patients after retrovirus-mediated gene therapy of SCID-X1. J Clin Invest 2008; 118:3132–42.
3. Stein S, Ott MG, Schultze-Strasser S, et al. Genomic instability and myelodysplasia with monosomy 7 consequent to EVI1 activation after gene therapy for chronic granulomatous disease. Nat Med 2010;16:198–204.

# Preface

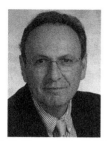

Chaim M. Roifman, MD, FRCPC, FCACB
*Guest Editor*

This issue of the *Immunology and Allergy Clinics of North America* contains contributions from leaders in the field discussing the option of hematopoietic stem cell transplantation (HSCT) for conditions other than severe combined immunodeficiency. Immunologists frequently face the dilemma of "To BMT or not to BMT." Each condition should be carefully studied, ideally with homogenous patient groups. Often such studies are not available. It is therefore imperative to set interim guidelines for transplantation. These could be based on several basic principles:

1. A diagnosis, preferably a molecular diagnosis has been established.
2. The condition has a high probability of reducing life expectancy (because of complications such as bleeding, chronic debilitating infections, or malignancy).
3. A condition with high burden of morbidity.
4. Hematopoietic stem cell therapy can cure the disease.
5. HSCT benefits outweigh risks of its associated complications.
6. There is no alternative superior treatment available at present.

Obviously, guidelines based on these principles should be periodically reassessed as novel treatments are introduced. A good example is the introduction of gene therapy for adenosine deaminase deficiency. Patients with this metabolic immunodeficiency have a poor outcome after HSCT from a donor other than a relative with an identical HLA typing. Gene therapy seems very promising (see the article by Cappelli and Aiuti elsewhere in this issue for further exploration of this topic) and could replace HSCT in these cases.

As the spectrum of indications for gene therapy in primary immunodeficiency expands, proper treatment guidelines will have to be established. The aforementioned principles used for HSCT are well suited to form the basis for these guidelines.

Chaim M. Roifman, MD, FRCPC, FCACB
Division of Immunology and Allergy
Department of Pediatrics, The University of Toronto
The Hospital for Sick Children
555 University Avenue, Toronto, ON M5G 1X8, Canada

E-mail address:
croifman@sickkids.ca

doi:10.1016/j.iac.2010.03.002
0889-8561/10/$ – see front matter
immunology.theclinics.com

# Purified Hematopoietic Stem Cell Transplantation: The Next Generation of Blood and Immune Replacement

Agnieszka Czechowicz, BS*, Irving L. Weissman, MD

**KEYWORDS**

- Hematopoeitic stem cell transplantation
- Nonmalignant hematolymphoid disorders
- Nonmyeloablative conditioning • Immune tolerance
- Autoimmune diseases

Severe combined immunodeficiency (SCID), systemic lupus erythematosus (SLE), and type 1 diabetes share one commonality: these diverse disorders can all be attributed to faulty immune effector cells largely caused by genetic mutations that alter hematopoietic cell-intrinsic function. These defective immune cells inherit their genetic deficiencies from hematopoietic stem cells (HSCs) as they differentiate. Thus, each of these unique diseases should be theoretically curable through the same strategy: replacement of patients' HSCs carrying the problematic mutation with normal HSCs from disease-free donors, thereby generating entire new, healthy hematolymphoid systems. Replacement of disease-causing stem cells with healthy ones has been achieved clinically via hematopoietic cell transplantation (HCT) for the last 40 years, as a treatment modality for a variety of cancers and immunodeficiencies with moderate, but increasing success. This modality has traditionally included

This investigation was supported by National Institutes of Health grants R01CA086065 and R01HL058770 (to I.L.W.). A.C. is supported by the Medical Scientist Training Program at Stanford University School of Medicine, as well as a grant from The Paul and Daisy Soros Fellowships for New Americans. The program is not responsible for the views expressed.
Affiliations that might be perceived to have biased this work are as follows: I.L.W. cofounded and consulted for Systemix, is a cofounder and director of Stem Cells, Inc, and cofounded and is a former director of Cellerant, Inc. A.C. declares no financial or commercial conflict of interest.
Institute of Stem Cell Biology and Regenerative Medicine, Stanford University School of Medicine, 279 Campus Drive, Stanford, CA 94305, USA
* Corresponding author.
*E-mail address:* aneeshka@stanford.edu

transplantation of mixed hematopoietic populations that include HSCs and other cells, such as T cells. This article explores and delineates the potential expansion of this technique to treat a variety of inherited diseases of immune function, the current barriers in HCT and pure HSC transplantation, and the up-and-coming strategies to combat these obstacles.

## ADVANTAGES OF PURIFIED ALLOGENEIC HEMATOPOIETIC STEM CELL TRANSPLANTATION

HSCs are the only cells within the body that at a clonal level have the ability to self-renew for life as well as give rise to all the different distinct mature effectors cells that comprise the blood and immune system.[1] These 2 properties give HSCs the sole responsibility for the proper lifelong maintenance of hematopoietic homeostasis. However, genetic abnormalities within HSCs can result in diseases such as immunodeficiency, autoimmunity, hemoglobinopathies, or hematologic malignancies, as these defects are passed down from the HSCs to their mature cell progeny, which then generate the diseased blood or immune system.

The first successful hematopoietic cell transplant involving reconstitution of an infant immunologic deficiency was accomplished by Good and colleagues in 1968.[2] Since then, HCT has been employed as an effective strategy to treat a multitude of hematolymphoid diseases. This procedure, more commonly known as allogeneic bone marrow transplantation, replaces mutant HSCs with functional ones from donor bone marrow grafts, which thereafter give rise to a complete normal hematolymphoid system that if stably engrafted persists for life.[3] Although allogeneic HCT can be an effective cure for most hematopoietic-intrinsic blood or immune diseases, it is rarely performed clinically except for life-threatening diseases and in near-death scenarios because of the toxicity of the procedure. Under current practices, allogeneic HCT has a transplant mortality rate of approximately 10% to 20%, far too high to justify its routine use in most nonmalignant settings.[4]

One of the most frequent and dangerous complications associated with allogeneic HCT is graft versus host disease (GvHD).[5] GvHD is a complex, immunologically mediated, host-directed, inflammatory response that is attributed to transplanted donor cells genetically disparate to their host. During GvHD, grafted mature T cells, having undergone tolerization on donor rather than host thymic epithelium, upon infusion into the host result in a violent immunologic response and particularly react against host lymphoid organs, skin, liver, and gut.[6,7] Although the likelihood and severity of GvHD can be minimized by transplantation from donors that are a close histocompatible match,[8] the risks and effects of GvHD remain unacceptably high and dramatically limit HCT.

Based on presentation of symptoms, GvHD has historically been classified into 2 distinct classes: acute and chronic. Acute GvHD is rapid, occurring within 100 days of HCT and presenting as a syndrome of dermatitis, enteritis, and/or hepatitis.[7] Chronic GvHD occurs at later time points and differs drastically from acute GvHD, often consisting of an autoimmune-like syndrome combining impairment of multiple organs or organ systems.[7] To these 2 commonly studied subsets of GvHD is added a third important subtype, subclinical but immunosuppressive GvHD (see later discussion).[9] Although T cells have been shown to play a dominant role in these severe complications of HCT, the exact molecular and cellular mechanisms underlying each subtype remain largely unknown.[10]

Despite a lack of complete understanding of the pathogenesis of GvHD, one potential solution to prevent its occurrence is to transplant purified HSCs. Often the terms hematopoietic stem cell transplantation (HSCT) and HCT/bone marrow transplantation (BMT) are used interchangeably in the literature, but in reality the clinical methodology differs dramatically. Although the efficacy of BMT relies on the activity of HSC, bone marrow is composed of a heterogeneous mixture of cells, including stem, multipotent progenitors, and mature blood cells, all of which are transferred to the patient in BMT. In contrast, HSCT refers to transfer of a highly purified population of strictly HSCs obtained from the donor bone marrow. The inclusion of cell populations other than HSCs and their resulting effects are what differentiate HCT/BMT from HSCT.

HSCs are defined as cells that can give rise to long-term multilineage reconstitution, as demonstrated when they are transferred into a hematolymphoid-depleted, irradiated host. Separation based on expression of discrete phenotypic cell surface markers and verification of their functionality in this manner led to identification and isolation of human[11] and murine HSCs.[1] HSCs are exceedingly rare cells, making up less than 0.1% of a bone marrow graft. Based on the efforts of multiple scientific groups, the HSC population has been prospectively isolated and refined to purity. All long-term HSC activity in adult mouse bone marrow is believed to be contained within a population marked by the composite phenotype of $c\text{-}Kit^+$, $Thy\text{-}1.1^{lo}$, lineage marker$^{-/lo}$, $Sca\text{-}1^+$, $Slamf1^+$, $Flk2^-$, and $CD34^{-}$.[1,12–16] Similarly, the phenotypic profile of human HSCs was validated to consist of $CD34^+$ and $Thy\text{-}1^+$, in addition to lacking $CD38^-$, $CD45RA^-$, and mature lineage markers.[11,17,18] Cells with these specific phenotypes are capable of giving rise to lifelong hematopoiesis on transplantation at the single mouse-cell level into congenic myeloablated mice,[17,19–21] and at the 10 human-cell level in xenogeneic models with myeloablated immunodeficient mice.[18] Validation of in vivo human HSC activity with cells of this phenotype was confirmed in several phase 1 clinical trials, which showed autologous HSC-rescued blood formation in myeloablated recipients and provided sustained, prolonged hematopoiesis.[22–24]

Isolation of HSCs based on the cell surface markers listed above can be accomplished by combining magnetic bead selection and fluorescence activated cells sorting (FACS) methods, yielding purified HSCs that are depleted of other polluting hematopoietic populations such as T cells.[1] Prospective isolation of HSCs in this manner is the only effective way to completely purge grafts of contaminating, unwanted populations from clinically transplantable HSC populations. In the case of autologous transplantation to treat malignancy, human HSCs purified in this manner provide long-term hematolymphoid repopulating activity and are free of contaminating resident or metastasized cancer cells.[22] However, in allogeneic transplantation for malignancies, HSC purification eliminates T cells that may function against the cancer and be responsible for the beneficial graft versus tumor (GvT) effect.[25]

In allogeneic HCT for nonmalignant diseases, purification of HSCs can be profoundly beneficial and can lead to significantly diminished procedure-related toxicity. Purified HSCT decreases the adverse outcomes of HCT/BMT; because removal of T cells from allografts completely eliminates GvHD.[26] Purification of HSCs from a graft eliminates the possibility of cotransplantation of host-reactive mature donor T cells, which are often contained within a graft and are primarily responsible for both acute and chronic GvHD.[10] In addition to the gross lesions associated with transplantation of T cells, low doses of T cells within a graft also contribute to underappreciated subclinical GvHD. In HCT, delays in immune reconstitution can be observed even in the setting where GvHD is not readily recognized, attributable to subclinical GvHD. Even after transplantation of grafts containing minimal contaminating T cells, donor T cells attack host lymphoid tissue and destroy tissue architecture, leaving the recipient vulnerable to opportunistic infections. Transplantation of purified HSCs eliminates subclinical GvHD and results in significantly accelerated immune reconstitution,[9] further increasing transplantation safety. As such, the complications and toxicities of BMT and HSCT are distinct, and further advocate for the transplantation of purified hematopoietic stem cells especially in nonmalignant settings.

## APPLICATION OF HSCT: CURING A VARIETY OF NONMALIGNANT HEMATOLYMPHOID DISEASES

Toxicity associated with HCT has dramatically restricted its current practice to life-threatening disorders such as hematologic malignancies and bone marrow failure states, where few other therapeutic options exist. However, HCT has other important potential applications beyond its current uses if HCT-associated toxicity could be eliminated. HCT has been shown to effectively reverse nonmalignant genetic hematologic disorders such as sickle cell anemia and β-thalassemia, as well as primary immune deficiencies,[27] if sufficient hematopoietic chimerism is achieved. In addition, early experimentation in rodents revealed that marrow transplantation could not only protect against irradiation death and prevent hematopoietic failure, but in the process could induce immune tolerance, resulting in the creation of hematopoietic chimeras that would accept skin grafts from the donor or host strain.[28] These and subsequent studies opened the opportunity to expand this technique as a therapeutic modality for a variety of immunologic diseases, and provided a potential alternative to lifelong administration of immunosuppressive drugs following organ transplantation—the aims of transplant biologists and clinicians now for over half a century.[29–32]

This phenomenon of permanent transplant tolerance is attributable to the elimination of donor-reactive T cells, primarily through negative selection in the thymus of developing T cells with donor-reactive antigen receptors. Transplantation of donor HSCs results in new immune cell generation on a chimeric microenvironment, leading to deletion of reactive immune effector cells against both host (via the thymic medullary epithelium) and donor (via donor derived thymic dendritic cells).[6,33] Recent studies illustrate that allotransplantation of purified HSCs either before or concurrent with transplantation of matched donor heart tissue precludes injury and subsequent rejection of donor organs.[34] Due to cotransplantation of either tissue organs and/or tissue stem cells with HSCs, long-term immune tolerance to donor tissues by the host can be achieved and the need for hazardous lifelong immunosuppression eliminated, as best illustrated in recent trials of kidney/bone marrow transplant patients.[30,35] The use of HSCT in this manner may significantly abrogate complications of solid organ transplantation, extending organ longevity and decreasing infection susceptibility. Future cotransplantation of HSCs and solid organ tissue generated in vitro from the same embryonic or induced pluripotent stem cell may be possible, expanding the pool of transplant candidates.

The concept of induced immune tolerance by HSCT can additionally be extended to the treatment of autoimmune diseases. HCT and HSCT have been demonstrated to have utility in blocking disease pathogenesis of a wide variety of autoimmune disorders such as diabetes mellitus type 1,[36] multiple sclerosis,[37] and SLE.[38,39] These autoimmune diseases are complex, multifactorial diseases often containing an environmental component; however, they also bear a genetic element and involve HSCs predisposed to generating self-reactive T-cell and/or B-cell clones that can react against and attack host tissues.[40] Transplantation of the disease can be achieved by transplantation of HSCs from donors predisposed to or bearing the disorder into otherwise healthy recipients.[41] Conversely, allogeneic transplantation of normal donor HSCs into diseased recipients generates tolerance and prevents attack of otherwise reactive tissues.

Cure of these diseases can be achieved by elimination of the host's reactive T cells, and subsequent generation of a new nonself-reactive T-cell compartment from the disease-resistant donor. Current transplantation procedures eliminate host immune cells and thus at least initially suppress the autoimmune disease, regardless of whether autologous or allogeneic HCT is performed. However, in these autoimmune disorders the HSCs are defective and predisposed to generating self-reactive immune cells, thus autologous transplantation as illustrated in mouse models of type 1 diabetes, allergic encephalomyelitis, and SLE is not curative. As such, syngeneic transplantation of purified HSCs in a mouse model of spontaneous autoimmune diabetes mellitus provides no long-term survival benefit.[41] Conversely, transplanted allogeneic HSCs are predisposed to generating nonself-reacting immune cells, and indeed in the same model completely prevent diabetes development throughout life.[41] Clinical data regarding autologous transplantation for autoimmune diseases is variable. In such settings, a naïve immune system is transplanted and, depending on environmental factors, may not always result in rapid re-creation of the diseased state. Some patients show excellent and long-lived clinical remission of disease, whereas others enjoy initial symptomatic benefit with subsequent relapse.[42]

Autologous transplantation reintroduces the host's defective HSCs, and therefore may not result in long-term cure. As the molecular basis for various monogenic hematolymphoid diseases is determined, gene therapy may become a realistic strategy to correct autologous HSCs before transplantation. On transplantation, these few modified HSCs could reconstitute a complete, corrected hematolymphoid system that persists for life. This strategy would be instrumental in the treatment of immune diseases, in addition to genetic and acquired nonmalignant blood diseases, such as sickle cell anemia for which currently allogeneic HCT is occasionally performed. In addition, gene therapy for HSCs may play a pivotal role in generating HSCs that produce immune cells predisposed to attacking tumors. However, to date gene therapy is individual specific, and is limited by the current inability to achieve reliable and rapid gene transduction with vectors that do not by insertional mutagenesis induce diseases such LMO2-activated acute lymphocytic leukemia.[43]

Furthermore, transplantation of HSCs generating mature cells resistant to infectious agents may prove an effective strategy to combat a magnitude of viral agents. Case reports of human immunodeficiency virus (HIV)-infected patients transplanted with HSCs from donors resistant to the disease resulted in at least preliminary cure of these patients. In these select scenarios, transplanted donor HSCs generated donor T cells bearing CCR5 defects, making them impenetrable to HIV.[44] Long-term outcome of these studies is unknown and the feasibility of such treatments using currently available transplantation strategies is questionable. However, these studies illustrate a potential new therapeutic use of HCT if other hurdles such as supply of resistant-matched donor cells are overcome.[45]

HCT has been repeatedly confirmed to be the singular curative therapy for this plethora of blood and immune diseases. To date, however, HCT has not been routinely applied in these manners to treat the hundreds of thousands of patients who suffer from these ailments, primarily because of concerns regarding the morbidity and mortality of allografting procedures. With elimination of GvHD by transplantation of purified HSCs that are debulked of reactive T cells, therapy of this nature may become a mainstream reality.

## BARRIERS TO EXPANSION OF HSCT

Continued improvements in the control of regimen-related toxicities are necessary to expand the applications of HCT. Current HCT methods hold exorbitant risk to the patient in terms of the transplant procedure–related morbidity and mortality, providing a major impediment to extrapolation of these practices to a multitude of conditions.

Although GvHD may be eliminated by transplantation of purified HSCs, much toxicity of HCT is also attributable to the conditioning regimens necessary to enable HSC engraftment. Current conditioning methods include irradiation and cytotoxic drugs such as high-dose chemotherapy, which can cause infertility, secondary malignancies, endocrine dysfunction, and organ damage.[46] Whereas in the malignant settings this conditioning serves the dual purpose of tumor eradication as well as preparation of the host, in the nonmalignant disease setting these regimens lead to inexcusable, nonbeneficial toxicity. Despite the ability of BMT/HSCT to cure many nonmalignant diseases, they have seldom been employed in the treatment of nonlife-threatening yet debilitating diseases, largely due to these associated risks. This situation necessitates the need for more specific and less toxic methods to allow efficient HSC engraftment.

Stable, robust chimerism is necessary in the treatment of these diseases, with disorders such as sickle cell anemia requiring approximately 20% chimerism to ameliorate the side effects of the disease.[47,48] In the absence of myeloablative therapy, this can be difficult to achieve.[49] In addition, engraftment of purified HSCs in the absence of other facilitator populations in the bone marrow poses an even larger engraftment challenge. Various facilitator populations that augment HSC engraftment, including in mice CD8 T cells or $CD8^+$ $TCR^-$ dendritic cells, have been identified in bone marrow; however, many of these cells may also contribute to GvHD and therefore their transplantation should be avoided.[50] Moreover, the identification and subsequent purification of non–T-cell facilitator populations in humans has not been executed, further limiting our ability to enhance the engraftment of HSC.

Historical clinical data have shown that T-cell depletion results in increased graft failure.[51,52] T-cell depletion is a major impediment to transplantation of purified HSCs, thwarting the current practice and consequently exposing patients to GvHD. Various "nonmyeloablative" protocols have been developed to permit engraftment of donor cells with attenuated conditioning regimens[53]; however, although these protocols are not completely myeloablative they are still nonspecific, ablate the bone marrow, and have severe regimen-related toxicities, instigating the need for better preparative regimens.

However, transplanting HSCs without traditional conditioning has been difficult.[54] Traditional myeloablative conditioning is thought to play a role in immune suppression as well as creating space for transplanted donor HSCs.[55] HSCs are thought to reside in specialized microenvironments in the bone marrow that can serve as fixed tissue niches for HSCs, thereby regulating HSC numbers and behavior. Although the precise identities of the niche cells are still largely unknown and controversial, there is a large amount of data indicating that HSC niches exist and are critical to HSC maintenance.[56]

HSCs require specific and special growth factors and cytokines to preserve their unique state. How they receive these signals has been a growing field of research and controversy. In 1978 Schofield[55] proposed that an HSC site-specific niche must exist to provide these signals and in this way oversee HSC numbers, by regulating an HSC's decision to undergo self-renewal, differentiation, or apoptosis. In a setting of finite numbers of such niches, transplantation of HSCs in excess of these spaces would be predicted to be futile; initial experimentation performed by Micklem and colleagues[57] supports this hypothesis. Others have since argued that space is not an important factor to donor HSC engraftment, and have shown that in unirradiated recipients, transplantation of whole donor bone marrow readily displaces endogenous host marrow. Rather than by specialized sites, the argument can be made that HSC number is regulated by availability of diffusible factors and thus conditioning need not be done to ensure HSC engraftment.[58–60] However, these experiments were performed with whole bone marrow, and the conclusions about broad HSC behavior and purified HSC engraftment ability must be taken into consideration in this context.

Using purified HSC transplants, the authors have recently shown that in normal and immunodeficient mice, at any one point only a small number of HSC niches are readily available for transplanted donor HSCs, and transplants without conditioning lead to very low donor HSC chimerism (0.5%).[61] Regardless of the number of HSCs transplanted, once the available HSC niches are saturated additional engraftment cannot be obtained.[62] Of importance, only HSCs can saturate these niches and cotransplantation of 1000 fold-excess of progenitors does not affect HSC engraftment, arguing that HSCs occupy discrete niches from their downstream progeny.[62] These data mimic those observed by clinical transplanters who, even in the absence of immune barriers, observe similar very low levels of donor HSC chimerism on transplantation of hematopoietic cells enriched for human HSCs into immunodeficient patients not receiving conditioning.[63] The low level of HSC engraftment in these patients is sufficient to restore immune function transiently through proliferation and expansion of immune progenitors; however, over time these few engrafted HSCs encounter exhaustion and loss of the graft is occasionally observed, thereby necessitating ways to increase initial HSC engraftment even in the immunodeficiency setting.[64]

Taken together, these studies suggest that in the absence of conditioning or facilitator populations, in both humans and mice donor HSC engraftment is limited by the availability of appropriate niches. Endogenous HSCs occupy appropriate, otherwise transplantable HSC niches, and therefore one strategy to enhance donor HSC engraftment may be to deplete host HSCs. The development of reagents that specifically displace host HSCs, rather than myeloablative conditioning techniques currently in use, could lead to safer transplantation-based therapies for hematological and nonhematological disorders.

## UP-AND-COMING STRATEGIES TO IMPROVE HSCT

HSCs are migratory cells.[65] Under homeostatic conditions they can be found in blood circulation in addition to bone marrow, albeit at very low but physiologically relevant frequency.[66] Recent studies have shown that HSCs enter the blood stream via division-independent egress from the bone marrow, leaving behind empty HSC niches available for transplantation, and explaining why low levels of engraftment are observed in nonconditioned settings.[66] HSCs continually egress from the marrow and enter the blood, suggesting that additional HSC niches may become available over time. Concordantly, saturation of engrafted HSC niches is transient and indeed, repeat rounds of HSCT transplantation lead to additional donor HSC chimerism.[61,66] This strategy may be one important path through which donor HSC engraftment can be increased with ease.

The natural vacancy of HSC niches admittedly is very slow, and therefore one proposed strategy to increase the competition between the donor and host HSCs is to augment the vacancy of the HSC niches through mobilizing endogenous host

HSCs out of their marrow microenvironments and into circulation. This goal may be accomplished with reagents such as AMD3100, which cause significant mobilization without noteworthy proliferation.[67] Limited murine studies have shown such drugs to function as effective nontoxic conditioning therapeutics.[68] However, even in the setting of HSC mobilization, transplanted donor HSCs must still compete with displaced host HSCs for HSC space. Therefore, alternative strategies to enhance engraftment by eliminating endogenous competing HSCs are desired.

HSCs rely on a variety of signals for survival and maintenance of their stem cell state. Specifically, HSCs have been shown to require continual c-kit ligand (SCF) for survival, and inhibition of this signal results in apoptosis.[69] The authors have recently shown that ACK2, an antagonistic monoclonal antibody to the murine c-kit receptor[70] in immunodeficient mice, eliminates murine HSCs and creates vacant HSC niches available for transplantation.[62] Donor HSC engraftment efficiency is significantly increased with such conditioning, without any toxic side effects other than transient graying (as c-kit is additionally present on melanocytes). Transplantation of high doses of HSCs or multiple rounds of ACK2 followed by HSCs result in very high levels of mixed chimerism (>90%).[62] Translation of such strategies, targeting human HSCs, may result in nonmyeloablative regimens that promote donor HSC engraftment with minimal toxicity, thereby significantly decreasing the morbidity and mortality currently experienced with present conditioning regimens.

Such novel conditioning strategies may be effective at obtaining high levels of HSC engraftment. However, conditioning methods including irradiation and cytotoxic agents not only play a role in the creation of incoming space for HSC, but additionally act as immune suppressants and play a role in immune-mediated HSC resistance. In immunodeficient patients, such novel "space-creating" strategies in conjunction with purification of HSCs may be sufficient to eliminate entirely the current toxicities associated with HCT. However, in immunocompetent settings additional reagents will need to be explored to inhibit the host's immune system, thereby preventing rejection of the incoming transplanted cells. T lymphocytes and natural killer (NK) cells classically are considered the primary immune mediators of allogeneic HSC resistance.[71] When transplant pairs are fully matched at the major histocompatibility complex (MHC) loci, T-cell immunity predominates. However, if MHC disparities exist, as in, for example, haploidentical transplantations, NK cells also play an important role. Thus, reagents to eliminate the engraftment barrier must deplete or significantly impair the function of both types of lymphoid cells. Monoclonal antibodies may play a significant future role, as they may be used to transiently deplete host T cells and host NK cells before donor cell infusion. Multiple immunosuppressive monoclonal antibodies to human lymphocytes currently exist, including anti-CD2, -CD52, -CD3, -CD4, and -CD8, facilitating the generation of purely antibody-based nontoxic conditioning.

## REVOLUTIONIZING HCT

Almost 60 years has passed since the early dismal but promising transplants performed by Thomas and colleagues,[72] and since then we have learned much about the biology of blood and immune transplantation. Yet today we still face many of the same hurdles faced by our predecessors, namely, the competing challenges of (1) complications arising from GvHD syndrome and (2) toxicities associated with preparative regimens necessary for cell engraftment.

Recent data suggest we may be bordering on developing therapies that overcome these obstacles. By combining these strategies, we may be at the tipping point of changing the practice and therefore application of HCT. If the strategies outlined in this article, or others in their stead, are employed successfully, we may witness a new exciting wave of HCT, and an expansion of the use of HCT from primarily for patients with rapidly lethal diseases to those with a variety of other hematolymphoid diseases for which HCT is currently unacceptable.

From the beginning of clinical HCT, immunodeficiency has been a good initial disease target because it allows for separation of the immune transplant barrier from the other transplantation obstacles, affording scientists and clinicians the ability to sequentially optimize individual treatment components. In this manner, SCID will likely be the first disease treated with the modalities outlined herein before they are extended to other applications. Moving forward, purified HSCT and novel conditioning strategies should allow for better treatment of SCID, obtaining higher donor engraftment without GvHD. Addition of antibody-based immunodepletion will subsequently allow for the combating of nonmalignant blood diseases. Thereafter, transplant tolerance may be achievable using such strategies as cotransplantation of HSCs and tissues/organs, and similarly, autoimmunity may be treated. The final goal is to treat patients whose organs have already been destroyed during autoimmune attacks, such as insulin-dependent type 1 diabetics lacking islet cells and, as has been shown in mice, concurrently transplant them with new organs as well as HSCs that impede rejection of the organ graft, prevent subsequent autoimmunity, and do not lead to GvHD.[41] Such dreams may become a reality in the distant future; meanwhile the incremental successes in any of these realms will allow for the gradual expansion of HCT as a therapeutic option for thousands of patients suffering from the diverse diseases of the blood and immune system.

## ACKNOWLEDGMENTS

The authors thank D. Bhattacharya and M. Howard for insightful review of the manuscript.

## REFERENCES

1. Spangrude GJ, Heimfeld S, Weissman IL. Purification and characterization of mouse hematopoietic stem cells. Science 1988;241(4861):58–62.
2. Gatti RA, Meuwissen HJ, Allen HD, et al. Immunological reconstitution of sex-linked lymphopenic immunological deficiency. Lancet 1968;2(7583):1366–9.
3. McCulloch EA, Till JE. The radiation sensitivity of normal mouse bone marrow cells, determined by quantitative marrow transplantation into irradiated mice. Radiat Res 1960;13:115–25.
4. Michlitsch JG, Walters MC. Recent advances in bone marrow transplantation in hemoglobinopathies. Curr Mol Med 2008;8(7):675–89.
5. Barnes DW, Loutit JF, Micklem HS. "Secondary disease" of radiation chimeras: a syndrome due to lymphoid aplasia. Ann N Y Acad Sci 1962;99:374–85.
6. Keever CA, Flomenberg N, Brochstein J, et al. Tolerance of engrafted donor T cells following bone marrow transplantation for severe combined immunodeficiency. Clin Immunol Immunopathol 1988;48(3):261–76.
7. Ferrara JL, Deeg HJ. Graft-versus-host disease. N Engl J Med 1991;324(10): 667–74.
8. Schierman LW, Nordskog AW. Influence of the B bloodgroup-histocompatibility locus in chickens on a graft-versus-host reaction. Nature 1963;197:511–2.
9. Tsao GJ, Allen JA, Logronio KA, et al. Purified hematopoietic stem cell allografts reconstitute immunity superior to bone marrow. Proc Natl Acad Sci U S A 2009; 106(9):3288–93.

10. Sprent J, Miller JF. Fate of H2-activated T lymphocytes in syngeneic hosts. II. Residence in recirculating lymphocyte pool and capacity to migrate to allografts. Cell Immunol 1976;21(2):303–13.

11. Baum CM, Weissman IL, Tsukamoto AS, et al. Isolation of a candidate human hematopoietic stem-cell population. Proc Natl Acad Sci U S A 1992;89(7):2804–8.

12. Kiel MJ, Yilmaz OH, Iwashita T, et al. SLAM family receptors distinguish hematopoietic stem and progenitor cells and reveal endothelial niches for stem cells. Cell 2005;121(7):1109–21.

13. Whitlock CA, Tidmarsh GF, Muller-Sieburg C, et al. Bone marrow stromal cell lines with lymphopoietic activity express high levels of a pre-B neoplasia-associated molecule. Cell 1987;48(6):1009–21.

14. Christensen JL, Weissman IL. Flk-2 is a marker in hematopoietic stem cell differentiation: a simple method to isolate long-term stem cells. Proc Natl Acad Sci U S A 2001;98(25):14541–6.

15. Matsuoka S, Ebihara Y, Xu M, et al. CD34 expression on long-term repopulating hematopoietic stem cells changes during developmental stages. Blood 2001; 97(2):419–25.

16. Adolfsson J, Borge OJ, Bryder D, et al. Upregulation of Flt3 expression within the bone marrow Lin(−)Sca1(+)c-kit(+) stem cell compartment is accompanied by loss of self-renewal capacity. Immunity 2001;15(4):659–69.

17. Osawa M, Hanada K, Hamada H, et al. Long-term lymphohematopoietic reconstitution by a single CD34-low/negative hematopoietic stem cell. Science 1996; 273(5272):242–5.

18. Majeti R, Park CY, Weissman IL. Identification of a hierarchy of multipotent hematopoietic progenitors in human cord blood. Cell Stem Cell 2007;1(6): 635–45.

19. Matsuzaki Y, Kinjo K, Mulligan RC, et al. Unexpectedly efficient homing capacity of purified murine hematopoietic stem cells. Immunity 2004;20(1):87–93.

20. Wagers AJ, Christensen JL, Weissman IL. Cell fate determination from stem cells. Gene Ther 2002;9(10):606–12.

21. Camargo FD, Chambers SM, Drew E, et al. Hematopoietic stem cells do not engraft with absolute efficiencies. Blood 2006;107(2):501–7.

22. Negrin RS, Atkinson K, Leemhuis T, et al. Transplantation of highly purified CD34+Thy-1+ hematopoietic stem cells in patients with metastatic breast cancer. Biol Blood Marrow Transplant 2000;6(3):262–71.

23. Vose JM, Bierman PJ, Lynch JC, et al. Transplantation of highly purified CD34+Thy-1+ hematopoietic stem cells in patients with recurrent indolent non-Hodgkin's lymphoma. Biol Blood Marrow Transplant 2001;7(12):680–7.

24. Michallet M, Philip T, Philip I, et al. Transplantation with selected autologous peripheral blood CD34+Thy1+ hematopoietic stem cells (HSCs) in multiple myeloma: impact of HSC dose on engraftment, safety, and immune reconstitution. Exp Hematol 2000;28(7):858–70.

25. Ito M, Shizuru JA. Graft-vs.-lymphoma effect in an allogeneic hematopoietic stem cell transplantation model. Biol Blood Marrow Transplant 1999;5(6): 357–68.

26. Shizuru JA, Jerabek L, Edwards CT, et al. Transplantation of purified hematopoietic stem cells: requirements for overcoming the barriers of allogeneic engraftment. Biol Blood Marrow Transplant 1996;2(1):3–14.

27. Barth E, Malorgio C, Tamaro P. Allogeneic bone marrow transplantation in hematologic disorders of childhood: new trends and controversies. Haematologica 2000;85(11 Suppl):2–8.

28. Main JM, Prehn RT. Successful skin homografts after the administration of high dosage X radiation and homologous bone marrow. J Natl Cancer Inst 1955; 15(4):1023–9.
29. Starzl TE, Demetris AJ, Murase N, et al. Cell migration, chimerism, and graft acceptance. Lancet 1992;339(8809):1579–82.
30. Scandling JD, Busque S, Dejbakhsh-Jones S, et al. Tolerance and chimerism after renal and hematopoietic-cell transplantation. N Engl J Med 2008;358(4):362–8.
31. Millan MT, Shizuru JA, Hoffmann P, et al. Mixed chimerism and immunosuppressive drug withdrawal after HLA-mismatched kidney and hematopoietic progenitor transplantation. Transplantation 2002;73(9):1386–91.
32. Alexander SI, Smith N, Hu M, et al. Chimerism and tolerance in a recipient of a deceased-donor liver transplant. N Engl J Med 2008;358(4):369–74.
33. Shizuru JA, Weissman IL, Kernoff R, et al. Purified hematopoietic stem cell grafts induce tolerance to alloantigens and can mediate positive and negative T cell selection. Proc Natl Acad Sci U S A 2000;97(17):9555–60.
34. Gandy KL, Weissman IL. Tolerance of allogeneic heart grafts in mice simultaneously reconstituted with purified allogeneic hematopoietic stem cells. Transplantation 1998;65(3):295–304.
35. Kawai T, Cosimi AB, Spitzer TR, et al. HLA-mismatched renal transplantation without maintenance immunosuppression. N Engl J Med 2008;358(4):353–61.
36. Nikolic B, Takeuchi Y, Leykin I, et al. Mixed hematopoietic chimerism allows cure of autoimmune diabetes through allogeneic tolerance and reversal of autoimmunity. Diabetes 2004;53(2):376–83.
37. van Gelder M, Kinwel-Bohre EP, van Bekkum DW. Treatment of experimental allergic encephalomyelitis in rats with total body irradiation and syngeneic BMT. Bone Marrow Transplant 1993;11(3):233–41.
38. Traynor AE, Schroeder J, Rosa RM, et al. Treatment of severe systemic lupus erythematosus with high-dose chemotherapy and haemopoietic stem-cell transplantation: a phase I study. Lancet 2000;356(9231):701–7.
39. Smith-Berdan S, Gille D, Weissman IL, et al. Reversal of autoimmune disease in lupus-prone New Zealand black/New Zealand white mice by nonmyeloablative transplantation of purified allogeneic hematopoietic stem cells. Blood 2007; 110(4):1370–8.
40. Todd JA, Bell JI, McDevitt HO. HLA-DQ beta gene contributes to susceptibility and resistance to insulin-dependent diabetes mellitus. Nature 1987;329(6140): 599–604.
41. Beilhack GF, Scheffold YC, Weissman IL, et al. Purified allogeneic hematopoietic stem cell transplantation blocks diabetes pathogenesis in NOD mice. Diabetes 2003;52(1):59–68.
42. Krauss AC, Kamani NR. Hematopoietic stem cell transplantation for pediatric autoimmune disease: where we stand and where we need to go. Bone Marrow Transplant 2009;44(3):137–43.
43. McCormack MP, Rabbitts TH. Activation of the T-cell oncogene LMO2 after gene therapy for X-linked severe combined immunodeficiency. N Engl J Med 2004; 350(9):913–22.
44. Hutter G, Nowak D, Mossner M, et al. Long-term control of HIV by CCR5 Delta32/ Delta32 stem-cell transplantation. N Engl J Med 2009;360(7):692–8.
45. van Griensven J, De Clercq E, Debyser Z. Hematopoietic stem cell-based gene therapy against HIV infection: promises and caveats. AIDS Rev 2005;7(1):44–55.
46. Ferry C, Socie G. Busulfan-cyclophosphamide versus total body irradiation-cyclophosphamide as preparative regimen before allogeneic hematopoietic

stem cell transplantation for acute myeloid leukemia: what have we learned? Exp Hematol 2003;31(12):1182–6.

47. Walters MC, Patience M, Leisenring W, et al. Stable mixed hematopoietic chimerism after bone marrow transplantation for sickle cell anemia. Biol Blood Marrow Transplant 2001;7(12):665–73.

48. Iannone R, Luznik L, Engstrom LW, et al. Effects of mixed hematopoietic chimerism in a mouse model of bone marrow transplantation for sickle cell anemia. Blood 2001;97(12):3960–5.

49. Storb R, Yu C, Sandmaier BM, et al. Mixed hematopoietic chimerism after marrow allografts. Transplantation in the ambulatory care setting. Ann N Y Acad Sci 1999; 872:372–5 [discussion: 375–6].

50. Gandy KL, Domen J, Aguila H, et al. CD8+TCR+ and CD8+TCR− cells in whole bone marrow facilitate the engraftment of hematopoietic stem cells across allogeneic barriers. Immunity 1999;11(5):579–90.

51. Kernan NA, Bordignon C, Heller G, et al. Graft failure after T-cell-depleted human leukocyte antigen identical marrow transplants for leukemia: I. Analysis of risk factors and results of secondary transplants. Blood 1989;74(6):2227–36.

52. Marmont AM, Horowitz MM, Gale RP, et al. T-cell depletion of HLA-identical transplants in leukemia. Blood 1991;78(8):2120–30.

53. Maloney DG, Sandmaier BM, Mackinnon S, et al. Non-myeloablative transplantation. Hematology Am Soc Hematol Educ Program 2002:392–421.

54. Tomita Y, Sachs DH, Sykes M. Myelosuppressive conditioning is required to achieve engraftment of pluripotent stem cells contained in moderate doses of syngeneic bone marrow. Blood 1994;83(4):939–48.

55. Schofield R. The relationship between the spleen colony-forming cell and the haemopoietic stem cell. Blood Cells 1978;4(1–2):7–25.

56. Morrison SJ, Spradling AC. Stem cells and niches: mechanisms that promote stem cell maintenance throughout life. Cell 2008;132(4):598–611.

57. Micklem HS, Clarke CM, Evans EP, et al. Fate of chromosome-marked mouse bone marrow cells transfused into normal syngeneic recipients. Transplantation 1968;6(2):299–302.

58. Saxe DF, Boggs SS, Boggs DR. Transplantation of chromosomally marked syngeneic marrow cells into mice not subjected to hematopoietic stem cell depletion. Exp Hematol 1984;12(4):277–83.

59. Stewart FM, Crittenden RB, Lowry PA, et al. Long-term engraftment of normal and post-5-fluorouracil murine marrow into normal nonmyeloablated mice. Blood 1993;81(10):2566–71.

60. Wu DD, Keating A. Hematopoietic stem cells engraft in untreated transplant recipients. Exp Hematol 1993;21(2):251–6.

61. Bhattacharya D, Rossi DJ, Bryder D, et al. Purified hematopoietic stem cell engraftment of rare niches corrects severe lymphoid deficiencies without host conditioning. J Exp Med 2006;203(1):73–85.

62. Czechowicz A, Kraft D, Weissman IL, et al. Efficient transplantation via antibody-based clearance of hematopoietic stem cell niches. Science 2007;318(5854): 1296–9.

63. Muller SM, Kohn T, Schulz AS, et al. Similar pattern of thymic-dependent T-cell reconstitution in infants with severe combined immunodeficiency after human leukocyte antigen (HLA)-identical and HLA-nonidentical stem cell transplantation. Blood 2000;96(13):4344–9.

64. Cavazzana-Calvo M, Carlier F, Le Deist F, et al. Long-term T-cell reconstitution after hematopoietic stem-cell transplantation in primary T-cell-immunodeficient

patients is associated with myeloid chimerism and possibly the primary disease phenotype. Blood 2007;109(10):4575–81.

65. Wright DE, Wagers AJ, Gulati AP, et al. Physiological migration of hematopoietic stem and progenitor cells. Science 2001;294(5548):1933–6.

66. Bhattacharya D, Czechowicz A, Ooi AG, et al. Niche recycling through division-independent egress of hematopoietic stem cells. J Exp Med 2009;206(12): 2837–50.

67. Broxmeyer HE, Orschell CM, Clapp DW, et al. Rapid mobilization of murine and human hematopoietic stem and progenitor cells with AMD3100, a CXCR4 antagonist. J Exp Med 2005;201(8):1307–18.

68. Chen J, Larochelle A, Fricker S, et al. Mobilization as a preparative regimen for hematopoietic stem cell transplantation. Blood 2006;107(9):3764–71.

69. Domen J, Weissman IL. Hematopoietic stem cells need two signals to prevent apoptosis; BCL-2 can provide one of these, Kitl/c-Kit signaling the other. J Exp Med 2000;192(12):1707–18.

70. Ogawa M, Matsuzaki Y, Nishikawa S, et al. Expression and function of c-kit in hemopoietic progenitor cells. J Exp Med 1991;174(1):63–71.

71. Murphy WJ, Kumar V, Bennett M. Acute rejection of murine bone marrow allografts by natural killer cells and T cells. Differences in kinetics and target antigens recognized. J Exp Med 1987;166(5):1499–509.

72. Thomas ED, Lochte HL Jr, Lu WC, et al. Intravenous infusion of bone marrow in patients receiving radiation and chemotherapy. N Engl J Med 1957;257(11): 491–6.

# Hematopoietic Stem Cell Transplantation and Other Management Strategies for MHC Class II Deficiency

Capucine Picard, MD, PhD[a,b,c],*, Alain Fischer, MD, PhD[c,d,e]

**KEYWORDS**

• Immunodeficiency • Antibody • Engraftment • Transplantation

Major histocompatibility complex (MHC) class II expression deficiency is a rare condition that results in primary immunodeficiency (MIM 209920). It is inherited as an autosomal recessive trait.[1] This disorder was first identified in 1978.[2] It is also frequently referred to as the (BLS). However, the term "bare lymphocyte syndrome" was first used to describe a defect in MHC class I expression in patients[3] and has been used synonymously for all defects involving expression of MHC class I (BLS type I), MHC class II (BLS type II), or both (BLS type III).[4] This article focuses only on the disorder that is associated with a defect in MHC class II expression and thus uses the term MHC class II deficiency. A deficiency in MHC class II expression leads to impaired antigen presentation by HLA-DR, HLA-DP, and HLA-DQ molecules on antigen-presenting cells (APCs), such as dendritic cells and macrophages.[5] This leads to combined immunodeficiency with defective CD4[+] T-cell development and a lack of T helper cell–dependent antibody production by B cells. MHC class II deficiency can be diagnosed by studying the cellular expression of MHC class II molecules, HLA-DR, on lymphocytes and monocytes. Patients with this disorder have no or a very low

[a] Study Center of Primary Immunodeficiencies, Necker Hospital, Assistance Publique-Hôpitaux de Paris, 149 rue de Sèvres, Paris 75015, France
[b] Laboratory of Human Genetics of Infectious Diseases, Institut National de la Santé et de la Recherche Médicale, U980, 156 rue de Vaugirard, Paris 75015, France
[c] University Paris Descartes, Necker Medical School, Paris 75015, France
[d] Institut National de la Santé et de la Recherche Médicale, U768, Necker Hospital, 149 rue de Sèvres, Paris 75015, France
[e] Unité d'Immuno-Hématologie Pédiatrique, Necker Hospital, Assistance Publique-Hôpitaux de Paris, 149 rue de Sèvres, Paris 75015, France
* Corresponding author. Study Center of Primary Immunodeficiencies, Necker Hospital, Assistance Publique-Hôpitaux de Paris, 149 rue de Sèvres, Paris 75015, France.
*E-mail address:* capucine.picard@inserm.fr

Immunol Allergy Clin N Am 30 (2010) 173–178
doi:10.1016/j.iac.2010.01.001
0889-8561/10/$ – see front matter © 2010 Elsevier Inc. All rights reserved.

level of MHC class II molecules detected on their B cells and monocytes. As for other combined immunodeficiency disorders, hematopoietic stem cell transplantation (HSCT) is currently the only available curative treatment for MHC class II deficiency.

## MHC CLASS II EXPRESSION DEFICIENCY AND GENETICS

The MHC locus itself is intact in patients with MHC class II expression deficiency. The lack of expression of DR, DQ, and DP MHC class II proteins on APCs is a result of impaired transcription of the MHC class II genes.[2] Previous somatic fusion experiments identified 4 complementation groups (A, B, C, and D).[6] Four disease-causing genes have since been identified and shown to encode regulatory factors controlling the transcription of MHC class II genes: CIITA for group A (MIM 600005),[7] RFXANK for group B (MIM 603200),[8] RFX5 for group C (MIM 601863),[9] and RFXAP for group D (MIM 601861).[10,11] The RFXANK, RFX5, and RFXAP proteins are all subunits of the ubiquitously expressed RFX complex. This complex binds directly to the promoters of all MHC class II genes and, together with other pleiotropic factors, forms the MHC class II enhanceosome. CIITA is an inducible factor that controls the expression of MHC class II genes expression by binding to the RFX complex and triggering transcription.

## MHC CLASS II EXPRESSION DEFICIENCY, CLINICAL MANIFESTATIONS, AND OUTCOME

More than 100 unrelated patients have been reported worldwide. Most patients are of North African origin (Algeria, Tunisia, and Morocco)[2,12,13] (Picard, unpublished data, 2010). Other patients have diverse ethnic backgrounds, including Israel, the Kingdom of Saudi Arabia, Pakistan, Turkey, France, Holland, Italy, Spain, and the United States of America.[2,12,14–16] Half of the reported cases have RFXANK deficiency (they belong to the complementation group B),[2] 75% of which are of North African descent (Morocco, Algeria, and Tunisia). A 26–base pair deletion disrupting a splice site has been found in 32 unrelated North African patients, indicating the existence of a founder effect[16] (Picard, unpublished data, 2010). The clinical course of disease, which is identical in the 4 groups, is characterized by the recurrence of bacterial, viral, fungal, and protozoan infections. Severe and chronic viral infections (eg, cytomegalovirus, herpes simplex virus, adenovirus, and enterovirus) are the hallmarks of this immunodeficiency and are associated with a poor prognosis. Recurrent bronchopulmonary infections caused by bacteria, viruses, and *Pneumocystis jiroveci* are particularly frequent. Protracted diarrhea, often leading to growth failure and severe hepatobiliary disease, is also common. Patients may also develop progressive hepatic failure caused by *cryptosporidium* infection. Infections start within the first year of life, and subsequent evolution of the disease is characterized by an inexorable progression of infectious complications until death ensues. Although some children reach puberty, and a few survive into adulthood, the majority die before the age of 10 years.

## MHC CLASS II EXPRESSION DEFICIENCY AND IMMUNOLOGIC FEATURES

The immunologic characteristics of MHC class II deficiency can be accounted for by the absence of antigen presentation via MHC class II molecules. Patients are unable to mount CD4[+] T-cell–mediated immune responses to specific antigens. Consistent with this, patient T cells do not show an in vitro response to antigens, which the patients had been immunized with or sensitized to by infection. Patients display T-cell lymphopenia, with a low CD4[+] T-cell count but a CD8[+] T-cell count that may be normal or low. The reduced number of CD4[+] T cells reflects the abnormal development of

CD4$^+$ thymocytes, resulting from defective MHC class II expression in the thymus. Surprisingly, however, the remaining CD4$^+$ T-cell population seems to be phenotypically and functionally normal.[17] Patient's CD4$^+$ T cells show normal alloreactive and proliferative responses to mitogens, but their potential function for physiologic responses are not known.[2] Although numbers of circulating B lymphocytes are normal, humoral immunity is severely impaired. Most patients have hypogammaglobulinemia, some with a reduced level of 1 or 2 immunoglobulin (Ig) isotypes, whereas some patients exhibit a hyper IgM profile. Patients do not show antibody responses to immunization and infection by microbial agents, except for a T-cell–independent antibody response against encapsulated bacteria. Autoantibodies associated with autoimmune disorders have been found in several patients. In conclusion, most patients are severely immunodeficient, with a low CD4$^+$ T-cell count and profound impairment of antigen-specific T- and B-cell responses.[2]

## MHC CLASS II EXPRESSION DEFICIENCY AND SUPPORTIVE TREATMENT

MHC class II deficiency has a poor prognosis, with a life expectancy of only a few years.[2,13] Only a minority of patients, characterized by a less severe clinical course, survives beyond the age of 20 years. There are no clear differences in prognosis among patients belonging to the 4 different genetic complementation groups. The leaky immunologic phenotype of some atypical patients is associated with a better outcome.[2] Treatment of infections and other complications can at best reduce the frequency and severity of the clinical problems that are associated with MHC class II deficiency. The optimal symptomatic care available to date involves the prophylactic use of antibiotics and administration of Ig with adequate nutritional support. Patients receive substitutive subcutaneous or intravenous Ig therapy (0.4 g/kg by 3 weeks). Regular Ig substitutive therapy results in a marked decrease in the number of bacterial infectious episodes. Patients also require antipneumocystis prophylaxis (trimethoprim-sulfamethoxazole, 25 mg/kg, 3 times a week). All live vaccines are strictly contraindicated in patients with MCH class II deficiency. A few patients have developed chronic lymphocytic meningitis caused by live attenuated poliovirus vaccination.[13] Finally, every effort should be made to detect viral replication in MHC class II–deficient patients who are candidates for HSCT (see later discussion).[18]

## MHC CLASS II EXPRESSION DEFICIENCY AND HSCT

HSCT is the only known treatment available to cure MHC class II expression deficiency. HSCT indication depends on clinical status (age, whether the patient is free from infection) and the availability of an HLA-compatible stem cell transplant donor.[18–20] Successful outcomes have been described, with narrow follow-up extending to more than 28 years.[18–20] European Registry data show that the survival rate associated with HSCT in patients with MHC class II deficiency is lower than that in patients with other forms of primary immunodeficiency.[18,20,21] This observation is independent of whether matched or nonmatched donors are used. HLA nonidentical transplantation (haploidentical or mismatched donors) for MHC class II immunodeficiency seems to be associated with a poor prognosis, with previous findings showing only 32% of patients to survive for more than one year after transplantation,[20] whereas 53% of patients receiving HLA-identical transplantation survived for more than one year.[18] A higher success rate seems to be achieved in patients undergoing HSCT before the age of 2 years.[19]

Moreover, MHC class II–deficient patients undergoing HSCT have increased risk to develop graft-versus-host disease (GvHD). Indeed, in the authors' experience among

15 patients with MHC class II deficiency, who had received transplants from an HLA-identical donor, the acute GvHD rate was 73%.[18] This rate was higher than GvHD rates reported for HSCT in patients with other primary immunodeficiency disorders.[20] The incidence and severity of GvHD seems to be correlated with the presence of ongoing viral infection before HSCT.[18] Aggressive antiinfectious therapy before HSCT, such as preemptive therapy against viral infections involving adenovirus, cytomegalovirus, or enterovirus, may therefore be beneficial in such patients. In conclusion, HSCT should be performed in MHC class II–deficient patients as early as possible, preferably before the age of 2 years. The best compatible donor available should be used. T-cell depletion of the transplant is required if the donor is not fully matched for HLA.

## MHC CLASS II EXPRESSION DEFICIENCY AND CONDITIONING REGIMENS

The myeloablation conditioning protocols used in MHC class II–deficient patients have been variable.[18–20,22–24] The most frequent protocol uses a combination of busulphan and cyclophosphamide.[20] Oral busulphan is given at a total dose of either 16 mg/kg or 20 mg/kg, depending on the period-related conditioning protocol and patient age, in combination with cyclophosphamide (200 mg/kg total dose). Most patients receiving a graft from an unrelated or HLA-mismatched donor are given in vivo immunosuppression treatment (using antithymocyte globulin, campath-IG, or anti-LFA-1 with or without CD2). GvHD prophylactic treatment involves administration of cyclosporin A, from the day before transplantation and continuing until day 180, with or without methotrexate. This GvHD prophylactic treatment is given in case of no T-cell depleted graft. Use of reduced-intensity conditioning protocols should be considered at least in patients with advanced disease.[25]

## IMMUNOLOGIC RECONSTITUTION AFTER HSCT

Most transplanted MHC class II–deficient patients with engraftment have normal cellular HLA class II DR expression. Low levels of HLA-DR cellular expression in several patients have been correlated with partial engraftment. MHC class II–deficient patients receiving transplants seem to display persistently low numbers of $CD4^+$ T cells. This finding is consistent with impaired thymic maturation caused by defective MHC class II expression on thymic epithelia. Despite $CD4^+$ T-cell lymphopenia, patients with complete or partial engraftment show normalization of antigen-specific T-cell stimulation and antibody production in response to immunization antigens. Of note, an impaired immune repertoire has been described for 2 patients with partial engraftment after HSCT.[23]

## SUMMARY

Five conclusions can be drawn from the authors' experience in the management of patients with MHC class II deficiency.[2] First, symptomatic treatment involves the prophylactic use of antibiotics, administration of Ig, and adequate nutritional support. Second, given the invariably fatal course of typical MHC class II deficiency and the poor outcome of HSCT performed after the age of 2 to 4 years, it is highly recommended that HSCT be performed in young children, using either an HLA-identical sibling or the best available compatible donor. Third, HSCT in MHC class II–deficient patients is complicated by a high incidence of acute GvHD associated with preexisting viral infections; every effort should be made to detect viral replication and treat these infections. Fourth, $CD4^+$ T-cells remain low in number (albeit, functional) in long-term survivors because of defective MHC class II expression by the thymic epithelial cells of the host. Finally, the lack of MHC class II expression in nonhaematopoietic cells does not seem to be detrimental for patients having undergone successful HSCT.

## REFERENCES

1. Notarangelo LD, Fischer A, Geha RS, et al. Primary immunodeficiencies: 2009 update. International Union of Immunological Societies Expert Committee on Primary Immunodeficiencies. J Allergy Clin Immunol 2009;124(6):1161–78.
2. Reith W, Lisowska-Grospierre B, Fischer A. Molecular basis of major histocompatibility complex class II deficiency. In: Ochs HD, Smith CI, Puck JM, editors. Primary immunodeficiency diseases. New York: Oxford University Press; 2007. p. 227–41.
3. Touraine JL, Betuel H, Souillet G, et al. Combined immunodeficiency disease associated with absence of cell-surface HLA-A and -B antigens. J Pediatr 1978;93(1):47–51.
4. Touraine JL, Marseglia GL, Betuel H, et al. The bare lymphocyte syndrome. Bone Marrow Transplant 1992;9(Suppl 1):54–6.
5. Mach B, Steimle V, Martinez-Soria E, et al. Regulation of MHC class II genes: lessons from a disease. Annu Rev Immunol 1996;14:301–31.
6. Benichou B, Strominger JL. Class II-antigen-negative patient and mutant B-cell lines represent at least three, and probably four, distinct genetic defects defined by complementation analysis. Proc Natl Acad Sci U S A 1991;88(10):4285–8.
7. Steimle V, Otten LA, Zufferey M, et al. Complementation cloning of an MHC class II transactivator mutated in hereditary MHC class II deficiency (or bare lymphocyte syndrome). Cell 1993;75(1):135–46.
8. Masternak K, Barras E, Zufferey M, et al. A gene encoding a novel RFX-associated transactivator is mutated in the majority of MHC class II deficiency patients. Nat Genet 1998;20(3):273–7.
9. Steimle V, Durand B, Barras E, et al. A novel DNA-binding regulatory factor is mutated in primary MHC class II deficiency (bare lymphocyte syndrome). Genes Dev 1995;9(9):1021–32.
10. Durand B, Sperisen P, Emery P, et al. RFXAP, a novel subunit of the RFX DNA binding complex is mutated in MHC class II deficiency. EMBO J 1997;16(5):1045–55.
11. Villard J, Lisowska-Grospierre B, van den Elsen P, et al. Mutation of RFXAP, a regulator of MHC class II genes, in primary MHC class II deficiency. N Engl J Med 1997;337(11):748–53.
12. Lisowska-Grospierre B, Fondaneche MC, Rols MP, et al. Two complementation groups account for most cases of inherited MHC class II deficiency. Hum Mol Genet 1994;3(6):953–8.
13. Klein C, Lisowska-Grospierre B, LeDeist F, et al. Major histocompatibility complex class II deficiency: clinical manifestations, immunologic features, and outcome. J Pediatr 1993;123(6):921–8.
14. Peijnenburg A, Van Eggermond MJ, Gobin SJ, et al. Discoordinate expression of invariant chain and MHC class II genes in class II transactivator-transfected fibroblasts defective for RFX5. J Immunol 1999;163(2):794–801.
15. Bejaoui M, Barbouche MR, Mellouli F, et al. [Primary immunologic deficiency by deficiency of HLA class II antigens: nine new Tunisian cases]. Arch Pediatr 1998;5(10):1089–93 [in French].

16. Wiszniewski W, Fondaneche MC, Lambert N, et al. Founder effect for a 26-bp deletion in the RFXANK gene in North African major histocompatibility complex class II-deficient patients belonging to complementation group B. Immunogenetics 2000;51(4–5):261–7.

17. Rieux-Laucat F, Le Deist F, Selz F, et al. Normal T cell receptor V beta usage in a primary immunodeficiency associated with HLA class II deficiency. Eur J Immunol 1993;23(4):928–34.

18. Renella R, Picard C, Neven B, et al. Human leucocyte antigen-identical haematopoietic stem cell transplantation in major histocompatiblity complex class II immunodeficiency: reduced survival correlates with an increased incidence of acute graft-versus-host disease and pre-existing viral infections. Br J Haematol 2006;134(5):510–6.

19. Klein C, Cavazzana-Calvo M, Le Deist F, et al. Bone marrow transplantation in major histocompatibility complex class II deficiency: a single-center study of 19 patients. Blood 1995;85(2):580–7.

20. Antoine C, Muller S, Cant A, et al. Long-term survival and transplantation of haemopoietic stem cells for immunodeficiencies: report of the European experience 1968–99. Lancet 2003;361(9357):553–60.

21. Fischer A, Landais P, Friedrich W, et al. Bone marrow transplantation (BMT) in Europe for primary immunodeficiencies other than severe combined immunodeficiency: a report from the European Group for BMT and the European Group for Immunodeficiency. Blood 1994;83(4):1149–54.

22. Saleem MA, Arkwright PD, Davies EG, et al. Clinical course of patients with major histocompatibility complex class II deficiency. Arch Dis Child 2000;83(4):356–9.

23. Godthelp BC, van Eggermond MC, Peijnenburg A, et al. Incomplete T-cell immune reconstitution in two major histocompatibility complex class II-deficiency/bare lymphocyte syndrome patients after HLA-identical sibling bone marrow transplantation. Blood 1999;94(1):348–58.

24. Bonduel M, Pozo A, Zelazko M, et al. Successful related umbilical cord blood transplantation for graft failure following T cell-depleted non-identical bone marrow transplantation in a child with major histocompatibility complex class II deficiency. Bone Marrow Transplant 1999;24(4):437–40.

25. Satwani P, Cooper N, Rao K, et al. Reduced intensity conditioning and allogeneic stem cell transplantation in childhood malignant and nonmalignant diseases. Bone Marrow Transplant 2008;41(2):173–82.

# Hematopoietic Cell Transplantation for Wiskott-Aldrich Syndrome: Advances in Biology and Future Directions for Treatment

Sung-Yun Pai, MD[a,b,c], Luigi D. Notarangelo, MD[c,d],*

**KEYWORDS**

- Wiskott-Aldrich syndrome • Chimerism
- X-linked thrombocytopenia
- Hematopoietic cell transplantation • Immunodeficiency

The Wiskott-Aldrich syndrome (WAS) is an X-linked disorder characterized by a triad of diagnostic clinical elements: immunodeficiency, eczema, and hemorrhage caused by thrombocytopenia with small-sized platelets. Manifestations of immunodeficiency in patients with WAS include recurrent and severe infections, autoimmunity, and malignancies. WAS was originally described in 1936,[1] but the X-linked pattern of inheritance was defined only 18 years later.[2] The gene responsible for disease, *WAS*, was cloned in 1994[3] and encodes a 502–amino acid protein (WAS protein [WASp])

Dr Pai receives support from the Translational Investigator Service Award from Children's Hospital Boston. Dr Notarangelo receives support from The Manton Foundation. This work was also supported by NIH grant P01-HL-059561-11A1 (to LDN).
<sup>a</sup> Division of Hematology-Oncology, Children's Hospital Boston, Karp Family Research Laboratories, 8th Floor, Room 8214, 1 Blackfan Circle, Boston, MA 02115, USA
<sup>b</sup> Department of Pediatric Oncology, Dana-Farber Cancer Institute, 44 Binney Street, Boston, MA 02115, USA
<sup>c</sup> Harvard Medical School, 25 Shattuck Street, Boston, MA 02115, USA
<sup>d</sup> Division of Immunology and The Manton Center for Orphan Disease Research, Children's Hospital Boston, Karp Family Research Laboratories, 9th Floor, Room 9210, 1 Blackfan Circle, Boston, MA 02115, USA
* Corresponding author. Division of Immunology and The Manton Center for Orphan Disease Research, Children's Hospital Boston, Karp Family Research Laboratories, 9th Floor, Room 9210, 1 Blackfan Circle Boston, MA 02115.
*E-mail address:* Luigi.Notarangelo@childrens.harvard.edu

Immunol Allergy Clin N Am 30 (2010) 179–194
doi:10.1016/j.iac.2010.02.001
0889-8561/10/$ – see front matter © 2010 Elsevier Inc. All rights reserved.

selectively expressed in hematopoietic cells, where it acts as a key regulator of the actin cytoskeleton.[4] *WAS* mutations that abrogate expression or function of WASp are responsible for WAS, whereas hypomorphic *WAS* mutations may also cause a milder form of the disease X-linked thrombocytopenia (XLT).[5] The latter, characterized by hemorrhages caused by thrombocytopenia associated with no or minor infections and eczema, is allelic to WAS.[5] The platelet count may significantly fluctuate, and hemorrhagic manifestations may be particularly mild, in patients with intermittent XLT.[6] In contrast, some missense mutations in the Cdc42-binding domain of WAS result in constitutive activation of the protein, causing X-linked neutropenia,[7–9] with neither thrombocytopenia nor signs of T-cell immunodeficiency. The phenotype of X-linked neutropenia is very different from that observed in WAS and XLT, and is characterized by increased apoptosis and defects of mitosis and cytokinesis[10] that may lead to myelodysplasia. The variability of clinical manifestations associated with null and hypomorphic *WAS* mutations has led to the development of a scoring system to grade the severity of the disease (**Table 1**).

Thrombocytopenia with small-sized platelets is the most consistent feature of the disease. Hemorrhages occur in greater than 80% of patients[11,12] and commonly include petechiae, epistaxis, and bloody diarrhea. Severe bleeding episodes (intestinal or intracranial hemorrhages) are also common (20%–30%) and cause death in 4% to 10% of patients.[11,12]

Bacterial (otitis media, skin abscesses, pneumonia, sepsis, meningitis) and viral (especially caused by herpes simplex and cytomegalovirus) infections are common, and are particularly severe in patients with WAS.[11] Several immunologic abnormalities contribute to the increased susceptibility to infections. Patients with WAS are unable to mount antibody responses to carbohydrate antigens,[13] and their response to protein antigens is also often impaired; in contrast, response to T-dependent antigens is typically normal in patients with XLT.[14] The inability to mount antibody responses to carbohydrate antigens and the increased susceptibility to invasive infections caused by blood-borne pathogens correlate with severe abnormalities of the marginal zone

**Table 1**
**Scoring system to grade the severity of clinical manifestations in patients with Wiskott-Aldrich syndrome and X-linked thrombocytopenia**

| | iXLT | XLT | | WAS | | |
|---|---|---|---|---|---|---|
| Score | <1 | 1 | 2 | 3 | 4 | 5 |
| Thrombocytopenia | -/+ | + | + | + | + | + |
| Small platelets | + | + | + | + | + | + |
| Eczema | - | - | (+) | + | ++ | (+)/+/++ |
| Immunodeficiency | - | -/(+) | (+) | + | + | (+)/+ |
| Infections | - | - | (+) | + | +/++ | (+)/+/++ |
| Autoimmunity or malignancy | - | - | - | - | - | + |

Scoring system: -, absent; (+), mild; +, present; ++, present and severe.

Patients who develop a score 5 are defined as 5A if they present autoimmunity, and 5M if they develop malignancies. Patients may change their score during their lifetime. In particular, patients with XLT may progress to WAS and may occasionally reach a score of 5.

*Abbreviations:* iXLT, intermittent X-linked thrombocytopenia; WAS, Wiskott-Aldrich syndrome; XLT, X-linked thrombocytopenia.

*Data from* Ochs HD, Filipovich AH, Veys P, et al. Wiskott-Aldrich syndrome: diagnosis, clinical and laboratory manifestations, and treatment. Biol Blood Marrow Transplant 2009;15(1 Suppl): 84–90.

of the spleen,[15] and similar findings have been reported in *Was*[−/−] mice.[16,17] Immuno-globulin abnormalities (low IgM, high IgA, and high IgE serum levels) are observed with similar frequency in patients with WAS and with XLT (Luigi D. Notarangelo, unpublished observation, 2010).[11] Defects of cell-mediated immunity, however, are more common and severe among WAS patients. In particular, T lymphocytes from patients with WAS fail to respond to immobilized anti-CD3 monoclonal antibody, show reduced proliferation to mitogens and antigens, and are impaired in their ability to secrete interleukin-2 and other Th1 cytokines upon in vitro activation.[18–20] In addition, patients with WAS show progressive T- and B-cell lymphopenia, but reduction of naive circulating T lymphocytes is apparent already early in life.[21] Defective cytolytic activity of natural killer cells may also contribute to increased frequency of viral infections,[22] and is more severe in patients with WAS than with XLT.[23]

Finally, monocytes and dendritic cells from patients with WAS show severe abnormalities of the actin cytoskeleton and impaired directional migration.[24] Defective interaction between dendritic cells and T lymphocytes may cause impaired T-cell priming, as also shown in the murine model of the disease.[25,26] Eczema is common (80%) in patients with WAS,[12] but less so (41%) in patients with XLT.[11] In addition to increased IgE serum levels[11] and skewed Th2 cytokine profile,[19] defective migration of Langer-hans cells has also been implicated in the pathophysiology of eczema.[27,28]

The incidence of autoimmune manifestations is markedly increased among patients with WAS, and ranges from 22% to 72% in various series.[11,12,29,30] Autoimmune hemolytic anemia, vasculitis, arthritis, nephropathy, and inflammatory bowel disease are particularly common. In addition, idiopathic thrombocytopenic purpura has been frequently observed in patients who develop a relapse of thrombocytopenia following splenectomy, and may even contribute to the pathophysiology of thrombo-cytopenia in unsplenectomized WAS patients.[31] Although the scoring system (see **Table 1**) dictates that patients with XLT do not have autoimmune manifestations at diagnosis, these may develop over time, and IgA nephropathy is particularly common (19%).[11] Occurrence of autoimmunity in WAS has prognostic implications and has been associated with reduced survival and higher risk of developing malignancies.[12,29] Multiple mechanisms may account for autoimmunity in WAS.[30,32] WASP-deficient natural regulatory T (nTreg) cells are severely impaired in their suppressive function.[33–35] Furthermore, patients with WAS and *Was*[−/−] mice have a reduced number and impaired function of invariant natural killer T (NKT) cells,[36,37] another population of cells with important immunoregulatory properties. Finally, impairment in the ability of dendritic cells to migrate in response to chemoattractants and to interact with T lymphocytes, and chronic immune activation resulting from inefficient pathogen clearance, may also play a role in the autoimmunity of WAS.[30]

Malignancies, predominantly lymphoma, leukemia and myelodysplasia, have been reported in 13%[12] and 22%[11] of patients in two series. They may occur in childhood, but are more frequent during adolescence or early adulthood, WAS patients are particularly susceptible to lymphoproliferative disease caused by Epstein-Barr virus (EBV).[38] It has been speculated that the increased occurrence of malignancy in patients with WAS is simply a late manifestation of the associated immunodeficiency. As the vast majority of malignancies seen are restricted to hematopoietic cells, where WASp is exclusively expressed, WASp-dependent hematopoietic cell-intrinsic abnormalities may also play an additional oncogenic role.

Initial reports indicated that median survival in patients with WAS is 20 years of age.[12] Death is mostly caused by hemorrhage, malignancy, and severe infection. Conservative management includes prompt and aggressive treatment of infections, immunoglobulin replacement therapy in patients with antibody deficiency, immunosuppressive drugs for autoimmune manifestations, surveillance for tumors, and anti-CD20 monoclonal antibody in patients with EBV lymphoproliferative disease. In the past, elective splenectomy has been used to reverse the thrombocytopenia, resulting in significant increase of the platelet count in up to 85% of patients. A significant fraction of patients (15%), however, develop chronic idiopathic thrombocytopenic purpura after splenectomy. Furthermore, splenectomy in WAS leads to increased risk of invasive pyogenic infections even in patients who receive antimicrobial prophylaxis. For this reason, many no longer consider splenectomy to be part of the routine therapeutic plan.[39]

Despite advances in diagnosis and clinical care, patients with severe disease (in particular, those who fail to express WASp) continue to have poor survival. In one recent study, the 20-year probability of overall survival was 0% for patients who fail to express WASp versus 92.3% among those who express reduced levels of normal-sized protein.[11] These data emphasize the importance of considering hematopoietic cell transplantation (HCT) in the treatment of WAS, especially for patients with more severe forms of the disease.

## MOLECULAR BASIS OF WAS AND GENOTYPE-PHENOTYPE CORRELATION ANALYSIS

Variability of the clinical and laboratory features among patients with *WAS* mutations has prompted genotype-phenotype correlation analysis. Polyclonal and monoclonal antibodies to WASp have been developed and used successfully for diagnostic and prognostic purposes.[40–42] Mutation analysis at the *WAS* locus has shown that most XLT patients carry missense mutations in exons 1 and 2 of the gene.[43] This corresponds to a region at the N-terminus of WASp that interacts with the WASP-interacting protein,[44] which stabilizes WASp.[45] Accordingly, patients with XLT who carry missense mutations in exons 1 and 2 of the WAS gene typically have reduced amounts of normal-sized WASp.[11,41,43] Occasionally, an XLT phenotype is also observed in patients who carry splice-site mutations, allowing for residual expression of full-sized transcript.[43] In contrast, a more severe WAS phenotype is generally associated with nonsense and frameshift mutations.[43] Mutation analysis alone is of limited value in predicting the clinical phenotype, since patients with WAS also may carry missense mutations (especially in regions other than exons 1 and 2) and some missense mutations in exon 2 are associated with a severe clinical phenotype. Analysis of WASp expression in lymphocytes has been used with great success in predicting the clinical phenotype. In a study of 50 patients with *WAS* mutations, positivity for WASp expression correlated with reduced incidence of severe infections, lower risk of mortality from intracranial hemorrhage, and prolonged survival.[11] It is important to note, however, that patients with XLT may progress to WAS with age, and may develop autoimmune complications and malignancies, albeit with reduced frequency and later in life than patients with WAS.

Finally, somatic mutations, many of which restore WASp expression, have been frequently observed in patients with WAS.[46] The higher frequency of revertants among T lymphocytes (especially CD8$^+$ T cells) indicates that WASp expression confers a stronger selective proliferation or differentiation advantage among such cells. These data are in keeping with in vivo observations in *Was*$^{+/-}$ mice, in which a striking predominance of WASp-expressing cells has been observed among peripheral T cells (especially CD8$^+$ and Treg lymphocytes), and among NKT lymphocytes and marginal zone B cells, but not among myeloid cells.[16,17] There is currently, however, no conclusive evidence that emergence of revertant clones in patients with WAS is associated with clinical improvement. Altogether, these observations suggest that expansion of certain

WASp-expressing cells can be expected in patients developing mixed chimerism, a tendency that may have important clinical implications for HCT and gene therapy.

## HCT IN WAS: A HISTORICAL PERSPECTIVE

The formal proof that HCT could cure WAS revealed a requirement for both immuno-suppression and myelosuppression; this remains the standard approach to curative therapy even today. Successful induction of high-level donor lymphocyte chimerism and development of isohemagglutinin antibodies 6 weeks after immunosuppression with 200 mg/kg of cyclophosphamide and HCT from an HLA-matched sibling was reported in 1968.[47] The patient remained thrombocytopenic, did not convert blood type to donor, and eventually died at 36 years of age secondary to complications of graft-versus-host disease following a second transplant preceded by myeloablative conditioning.[48] Correction of hematopoiesis in patients with WAS requires myelosup-pression in addition to immunosuppression, as demonstrated in 1978 by Parkman and colleagues.[49] They reported two patients who achieved normalization of hematologic and immunologic abnormalities after HCT with the use of anti–human thymocyte serum and total body irradiation (one patient also received procarbazine). Within a few years, two reports showed that myeloablative doses of busulfan and immuno-suppression with cyclophosphamide also corrected the disease.[50,51] This regimen has been the standard preparative backbone for HCT for WAS, and indeed for most nonmalignant disease.

Initially, HCT for WAS was mostly restricted to patients for whom an HLA-identical sibling was available. The demonstration that in vitro T-cell–depleted grafts from HLA-mismatched family donors (parents) could successfully reconstitute immunity in patients with severe combined immune deficiency (SCID)[52,53] led investigators to explore a similar approach for WAS. Results, however, have been disappointing. An early report from Memorial Sloan-Kettering showed only one of six patients surviving; two patients had graft rejection despite total body irradiation–based conditioning and EBV-positive lymphoma, whereas three developed graft-versus-host disease.[54] Summary data from the pooled European experience show 45% survival of 43 patients undergoing parental transplant compared with 81% survival of 32 patients undergoing sibling matched transplant.[55] Unlike patients with SCID, who lack T-cell function entirely, patients with WAS, even when heavily immunosuppressed, appar-ently resist engraftment in the T cell–depleted setting. Given these poor outcomes and difficulties in particular with posttransplant EBV-driven lymphoproliferative disease, T replete unrelated donor bone marrow transplants have been performed with greater frequency in the last decade (**Fig. 1**).

## CURRENT SURVIVAL AFTER MYELOABLATIVE HCT

The rarity of WAS and the variety of donor sources used (matched-sibling, matched- and mismatched-unrelated adult HSC, haploidentical-related, and matched and mis-matched cord blood) necessitate cooperative registry studies to analyze even straight-forward outcomes, such as survival. The European registry reported outcomes of 444 patients with non-SCID immunodeficiency enrolled from 1968 to 1999, of whom 103 patients had WAS with 62% overall 3-year survival.[55] Analysis of the full non-SCID cohort clearly demonstrated that matched-sibling donors fared best with 3-year survival of 71% versus 59% and 42% for matched-mismatched unrelated donor and mismatched-related, respectively.[55] This result was mirrored in the smaller WAS cohort with 81% of 32 matched-sibling donor recipients surviving versus 45% of 43 mismatched-related recipients surviving.[55] A study of the International Bone Marrow Transplant Registry

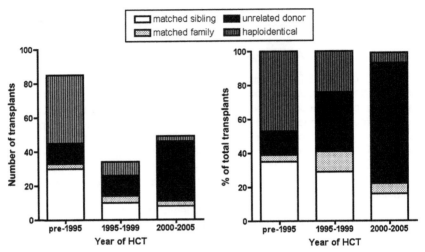

**Fig. 1.** Hematopoietic cell transplants for Wiskott-Aldrich syndrome in the SCETIDE Registry. The absolute number (*left*) and percentages (*right*) of HCT performed for WAS using different donor types (genotypically identical matched sibling, *white*; phenotypically identical matched family member, *speckled*; unrelated donor, *black*; mismatched haploidentical family member, *gray striped*) as reported to the SCETIDE Registry for the indicated time periods is shown. (*Courtesy of* Andrew Gennery and colleagues on behalf of the SCETIDE Registry.)

surveying outcomes of patients from a similar timeframe, overlapping with the European cohort, confirmed that matched-sibling recipients had a superior 5-year survival (87% of 55 patients) compared with mismatched-related recipients (52% of 48 patients).[56] These data were also independently confirmed in other smaller reports.[54,57,58] Unlike the good to excellent outcomes of mismatched-related transplants reported for SCID,[55,59] poor outcomes following this approach for WAS have led many centers to favor unrelated donors for patients who lack a family match.

The use of closely matched-unrelated donors for WAS rose dramatically during the 1990s; of 67 patients included in the survey of the International Bone Marrow Transplant Registry, 35 (53%) were transplanted from 1990 to 1993, and 29 (43%) from 1994 to 1996. This trend has continued in Europe as shown in **Fig. 1**, depicting both the percentage and absolute numbers of unrelated donor transplants reported to the SCETIDE registry before 1995, from 1995 to 1999, and 2000 to 2005. For these time periods 12, 12, and 35 patients underwent unrelated donor transplants, respectively, and because the number of mismatched-related transplants decreased, the percentage of unrelated donor transplants from 2000 to 2005 was 71% (Gennery and colleagues, unpublished data, 2010). This increase in unrelated donor transplants likely reflects both the increasing availability of alternative donors through expansion of the bone marrow donor international registry, and evidence from the Center for International Blood and Marrow Transplant Research (CIBMTR) study, which demonstrated that the survival of 52 boys with WAS undergoing unrelated donor bone marrow transplant at less than 5 years old was nearly identical to that of 55 boys undergoing matched-sibling bone marrow transplant (87% for matched-sibling; relative risk of death for unrelated donor <5 years, 1.34). Furthermore, advances in high-resolution typing of HLA alleles have resulted in progressive improvement of donor-recipient matching, and hence optimal selection of unrelated donors. An international survey of 73 centers caring for WAS patients in 2002 revealed that not all centers, particularly smaller ones, offered early HCT for WAS patients, but that 77.7% of larger centers routinely offered unrelated donor HCT.[60]

Experience with cord blood transplantation is accumulating, although very little summary data are available. The first reports of outcome after cord blood transplant for various disorders including WAS were published in 2000 by Knutsen and Wall[61] (one patient of eight in this series had WAS) and Thomson and colleagues[62] (1 patient of 30 with WAS). At least 29 other cases are known from the literature, many reported in aggregate with other diagnoses,[57,63–72] and one interesting report details the case of a boy treated with two separate unrelated cord blood units infused 8 days apart.[73] The largest report from Japan described 57 patients with WAS, of whom 15 underwent cord blood transplant with 80% 5-year survival (12 of 15), similar to both unrelated donor recipients (17 [80%] of 21) and matched-sibling donor recipients (9 [82%] of 11) from the same cohort.[57] Overall survival in these smaller series seems very good, in line with preliminary data from the CIBMTR showing 75% 3-year survival in 65 patients transplanted with cord blood under 5 years of age.[74]

Overall, studies on outcome of HCT for WAS suffer from limitations caused by the long period required to collect sufficient numbers. They fail to capture the effect of incremental changes in clinical care and improved high-resolution HLA typing that have impacted on transplant outcome. In the current era, except for historically poor outcome of haploidentical transplantation, comparative data are not yet mature to draw firm conclusions about the relative merits of donor match or stem cell source.

## IMMUNE FUNCTION AND HEMATOPOIETIC CORRECTION AFTER HCT

Complete donor chimerism cures the life-threatening manifestations of WAS, including hemorrhage, infection, autoimmunity, and malignancy, and can be achieved using myeloablative doses of busulfan in combination with cyclophosphamide or fludarabine, to facilitate robust and stable donor cell chimerism.[75] Mixed chimerism has been often reported following HCT for WAS, however, even when a myeloablative conditioning regimen is used.[76,77] Several groups have made use of reduced-intensity conditioning regimens to reduce drug-related toxicity in WAS patients who had significant pretransplant complications.[39,66,78,79] Typically, the use of reduced-intensity conditioning regimens for WAS results in mixed-split chimerism, where a variable proportion of lymphoid (especially T lymphocytes) cells are of donor origin, whereas myeloid cells remain mostly of recipient origin. Preferential engraftment or expansion of donor T lymphocytes has also been seen in studies of naturally occurring gene revertants,[46] human carriers,[41] and heterozygous $Was^{+/-}$ mice,[17] overall supporting the notion that the selective advantage conferred by normal WASp protein is lineage specific. In particular, it is well known that T cells from carriers of *WAS* mutations display a nonrandom pattern of X-chromosome inactivation, independent of the severity of the *WAS* gene mutation, whereas myeloid cells (and to a lesser degree B lymphocytes) from carriers of XLT do contain a fraction of WASp$^{dim}$ cells.[41,80] Similarly, a stronger selective advantage for WASp$^{+}$ cells within T lymphocytes than in other blood lineages also has been observed in $Was^{+/-}$ mice.[17] Finally, accumulation of WASp$^{+}$ T cells has been frequently reported in WAS patients, caused by somatic second-site mutations or true reversion events that restore WASp expression; in contrast, few examples are known of gene reversion in B or NK lymphocytes, and no cases of reversion in myeloid cells have ever been reported in WAS.[46,81]

Overall, these observations suggest that WASp-expressing cells should have a selective advantage in WAS patients developing mixed chimerism after HCT.

Indeed, this advantage in transplanted WAS patients is clearest in the T lineage, and is associated with significant clinical improvement, but not full correction of all aspects of the disease if high level myeloid chimerism is not achieved. Initial attempts at matched-related HCT for WAS resulted in donor T cells alone, with cure of T-dependent clinical manifestations, such as eczema.[49] The percentage of WASp-expressing lymphocytes in six patients with mixed chimerism reported by Yamaguchi and colleagues[77] was clearly higher at every time point measured than the percentage in monocytes, and donor chimerism was higher within CD8 than within CD4 T cells. After myeloablative transplant, 6 out of 21 patients at a single institution who had evaluation of T, B, and monocyte WASp expression had less than 100% donor chimerism, and in five of six, T-lineage chimerism was higher than monocyte chimerism. Two patients who had autologous reconstitution in the myeloid lineage, with relapse of thrombocytopenia, nevertheless retained 40% to 43% of T cells expressing WASp.[58]

Severe abnormalities of nTreg and NKT cells, two populations with important immunoregulatory properties, have been observed in patients with WAS and $Was^{-/-}$ mice and likely contribute to the autoimmunity of the disease.[33–37] A striking selective advantage for WASp expressing nTreg and NKT cells has been demonstrated in a competitive setting both in humans and mice.[33,37] It follows that engraftment of donor-derived nTreg and NKT cells may result in amelioration or even disappearance of autoimmunity in WAS patients who develop mixed chimerism after HCT. Data from a large European study show that autoimmune manifestations are a common complication after HCT for WAS, however, and are particularly frequent in patients who develop mixed chimerism.[76] Ascertaining the relationship between cell type–specific chimerism and autoimmunity is necessarily difficult given the overlap between autoimmune and alloimmune phenomena post-HCT, and requires further study.

Based on the current literature, loss of myeloid chimerism need not be accompanied by loss of T chimerism, and a minimal (yet, not well defined) threshold of myeloid chimerism must be maintained to prevent recurrence of clinically significant thrombocytopenia. It remains unclear what degree of donor chimerism is sufficient to prevent long-term complications of WAS, particularly autoimmunity. The kinetics and stability of donor chimerism in those with mixed or split chimerism is also unclear. These questions are the subject of a multi-institutional study of a large series of WAS patients posttransplant currently under analysis (Moratto and colleagues, unpublished data).

## SELECTION OF PATIENTS FOR HCT

Because of the heterogeneity of clinical phenotype in patients with WAS and variable outcome post-HCT depending on such factors as age and degree of HLA match, deciding which patients should be transplanted is not entirely straightforward. Certain subsets of WAS patients have excellent survival after HCT. The requirement for full myeloablation to achieve the greatest likelihood of full donor chimerism and freedom from autologous reconstitution, however, necessarily puts some patients at risk of early transplant-related mortality. There is only one comparative study of outcomes after supportive care versus transplantation, published in 1993.[82] This retrospective review of 62 patients showed that 18 of 31 splenectomized patients were alive, versus 14 of 19 undergoing HCT (12 of 12, 1 of 4, and 1 of 3 following matched-sibling, parental, and unrelated donor transplants, respectively). In the absence of more modern comparative studies that capture the impact of either therapy on long-term complications, the decision to take on the acute and chronic toxicities of transplantation at present should be made in the context of known predictors of poor outcome with supportive care alone.

The combination of clinical score and WASp expression allows for informative genotype-phenotype correlation that strongly supports early transplantation for certain patients. The presence of autoimmunity, particularly autoimmune hemolytic anemia or thrombocytopenia (manifested as failure to maintain platelet counts over 20,000 after splenectomy) is associated with a twofold to threefold risk of poor prognosis.[29] Patients achieving a clinical score of 5 because of autoimmunity (or malignancy) are at high risk and should be transplanted. Data to support transplantation based on WASp expression status come from Imai and colleagues.[11] This retrospective comparison of 27 WASp-positive and 23 WASp-negative patients in Japan showed that absence of WASp expression correlated best with measures of infection, particularly opportunistic infection; bacterial infection was four times more likely in WASp-negative patients compared with WASp-positive patients, and fungal and *Pneumocystis* infection was exclusively seen in WASp-negative patients. The retrospective nature of this study is subject to ascertainment bias, but nevertheless this study showed that the 10-year probability of survival was significantly lower in WASP negative patients (17 [76%] of 23 vs 26 [92.3%] of 27), even including 11 of 12 patients who survived after HCT.[11] These data suggest that patients with a clinical score of 3 (recurrent bacterial infections) or 4 (severe infection, including opportunistic infection) are likely to be WASp-negative, and that patients with scores of 4 or 5 regardless of WASp expression status should be transplanted with the best possible donor at an early age. Because survival after matched-sibling or well-matched unrelated donor HCT in patients under 5 years of age seems to be equivalent in large summary data,[56] a young WASp-negative patient with a well-matched donor with a score of 1 or 2 should also be strongly considered for early HCT before the age of 5.

Predictors that guide the decision to transplant XLT patients, who generally are WASp-positive, with normal or reduced levels of full-length protein, and who generally do not have clinical features meriting a score of 3 or above, are distinctly lacking. Although most such patients seem to be protected from malignancy, anecdotal reports of family members suffering from lymphoma exist.[11] Some patients do develop autoimmunity, and the presence or absence of WASp fails to segregate with autoimmune disease. Indeed, vasculitis, arthritis, autoimmune hemolytic anemia, and IgA nephropathy are all reported in WASp-positive patients.[11] Biomarkers to determine which XLT patients go on to have autoimmunity do not yet exist. Routinely available tests of immunologic function are also surprisingly lacking in sensitivity and specificity, because many patients with WAS and even lacking WASp protein have normal lymphocyte numbers, proliferation to mitogens, and total immunoglobulin levels, and a few may even demonstrate specific antibody responses to carbohydrate antigens.[12] HCT for XLT patients with clinical scores of 1 to 2, with WASp expression, should generally be limited to those with a matched-sibling donor, and alternative donor transplantation considered only for those with severe transfusion-dependent thrombocytopenia or intracranial hemorrhage.

For those patients with high clinical scores, relative contraindications to HCT include older age at transplant or pre-existing organ damage, such as lung disease, particularly if only mismatched donors are available. The propensity of WAS patients to develop mixed chimerism even after fully myeloablative busulfan and cyclophosphamide predicts that reduced-intensity conditioning may result in recipient-dominated mixed chimerism or autologous reconstitution. For this category of patients, somatic gene therapy, which has been successfully used in mouse models and in human cells,[83] can be considered. In light of the relative resistance to replacement of the niche by WASp normal hematopoietic stem cells (HSC), however, full myeloablation might not be avoidable and will be used in some of the trials currently planned (Adrian Thrasher and Marina Cavazzana-Calvo, personal communications, 2010).

## SUMMARY

Since the first transplant to treat WAS in 1968, there has been enormous progress in the understanding of WAS, namely the identification of the causative gene; characterization of the protein and its function; the discovery that XLT is also caused by mutations in WASp; and demonstration of a strong, yet incomplete, genotype-phenotype correlation. Likewise, studies of knockout mice, human carriers, natural revertants, and patients post-HCT have revealed intriguing biology about cell type–specific functions of WASp. In the post-HCT setting, development and survival of WASp positive cells in particular lineages, especially the T lineage, is favored.

Important progress has been made with regard to survival. Allogeneic HCT experience has matured and outcomes have improved as advanced pediatric intensive care, parenteral nutrition, and an expanded antimicrobial armamentarium have all become widely available. Allogeneic HCT for WAS has evolved from a specialized experimental technique reserved for a few patients, to a standard curative therapy to be considered immediately at the time of diagnosis. That well-matched unrelated donor HCT in young patients results in similar survival to those receiving sibling grafts has encouraged the use of HCT to the near exclusion of previously popular supportive measures, such as splenectomy. Indeed, because well-reconstituted WAS patients post-HCT who were previously splenectomized are nevertheless at risk of severe infections, including fatal sepsis,[58,76] the authors recommend that splenectomy be reserved only for patients who are unlikely ever to be transplanted.

In turn, there may be fewer and fewer patients for whom transplantation is relatively contraindicated; historically negative predictive factors may no longer portend poor outcome. The availability of sensitive testing for EBV and growing experience with anti-CD20 antibody has revolutionized prevention and treatment of EBV lymphoproliferative disease, such that the once uniformly dismal outcome of haploidentical HCT for treatment of WAS may have improved significantly.[84] The growing use of cord blood transplantation has expanded donor availability, although the effects of this new donor source and of improvements in HLA matching on outcomes remain to be measured. Whether the previously reported favorable effect of transplanting at a young age on survival will persist in light of these advances also must be reassessed in future studies.

Management of XLT remains controversial. Although several groups consider HCT from matched-related donors an option for XLT patients who are severely thrombocytopenic, this strategy is not unanimously accepted, and use of alternative donors is even more controversial in this setting. Progress in this area is hampered by the lack of prospective studies of long-term outcome in large cohorts of untransplanted XLT patients. Defining biomarkers that predict which XLT patients are at risk for late complications, such as lymphoma or refractory autoimmunity, may in turn identify those for whom the merits of early transplantation outweigh the upfront and late toxicities of allogeneic HCT. On the other hand, a large international retrospective study has recently been published[85], and confirms excellent long-term survival, but also a high probability of disease-related complications, for this group of patients.

The current short- and long-term toxicities of HCT are the main stumbling block for the ability to cure every patient with WAS and XLT, and much remains to be done. Indeed, the substance of the treatment itself has changed little. The standard conditioning strategy of busulfan and cyclophosphamide is the same as in 1981. Although this approach leads to full donor engraftment in most cases, a moderate proportion of patients develop mixed chimerism. This is even more common when reduced-intensity regimens are used to diminish drug-related toxicity. A number of questions remain. What is the minimum level of donor chimerism in the HSC or myeloid compartment required to maintain safe platelet levels post-HCT? How stable is donor chimerism over the long-term and can one predict who maintains or loses chimerism? Is mixed chimerism in the T compartment, particularly in nTreg or NKT cell lineages, sufficient to control autoimmunity? What degree of donor chimerism is sufficient to prevent malignancy? A multi-institutional retrospective study exploring these questions is nearly complete, but ultimately rigorous prospective long-term studies of cell type–specific chimerism and clinical outcome are required to answer these questions. Similarly, the efficacy of any novel conditioning approaches used to improve on the toxicity profile of busulfan and cyclophosphamide must be interpreted in relation to the desired level of chimerism to be achieved in each compartment. Continued multi-institutional and international collaboration to study this rare but fascinating disorder are needed to answer these questions.

## REFERENCES

1. Wiskott A. Familiärer, angeborener Morbus Werlhofii? [Familial, congenital Werlhof's disease?] Monatsschr Kinderheilkd 1937;68:212–6 [in German].
2. Aldrich RA, Steinberg AG, Campbell DC. Pedigree demonstrating a sex-linked recessive condition characterized by draining ears, eczematoid dermatitis and bloody diarrhea. Pediatrics 1954;13(2):133–9.
3. Derry JM, Ochs HD, Francke U. Isolation of a novel gene mutated in Wiskott-Aldrich syndrome. Cell 1994;78(4):635–44.
4. Thrasher AJ, Burns S, Lorenzi R, et al. The Wiskott-Aldrich syndrome: disordered actin dynamics in haematopoietic cells. Immunol Rev 2000;178:118–28.
5. Villa A, Notarangelo L, Macchi P, et al. X-linked thrombocytopenia and Wiskott-Aldrich syndrome are allelic diseases with mutations in the WASP gene. Nat Genet 1995;9(4):414–7.
6. Notarangelo LD, Mazza C, Giliani S, et al. Missense mutations of the WASP gene cause intermittent X-linked thrombocytopenia. Blood 2002;99(6):2268–9.
7. Ancliff PJ, Blundell MP, Cory GO, et al. Two novel activating mutations in the Wiskott-Aldrich syndrome protein result in congenital neutropenia. Blood 2006; 108(7):2182–9.
8. Beel K, Cotter MM, Blatny J, et al. A large kindred with X-linked neutropenia with an I294T mutation of the Wiskott-Aldrich syndrome gene. Br J Haematol 2009; 144(1):120–6.
9. Devriendt K, Kim AS, Mathijs G, et al. Constitutively activating mutation in WASP causes X-linked severe congenital neutropenia. Nat Genet 2001;27(3):313–7.
10. Moulding DA, Blundell MP, Spiller DG, et al. Unregulated actin polymerization by WASp causes defects of mitosis and cytokinesis in X-linked neutropenia. J Exp Med 2007;204(9):2213–24.
11. Imai K, Morio T, Zhu Y, et al. Clinical course of patients with WASP gene mutations. Blood 2004;103(2):456–64.
12. Sullivan KE, Mullen CA, Blaese RM, et al. A multiinstitutional survey of the Wiskott-Aldrich syndrome. J Pediatr 1994;125(6 Pt 1):876–85.
13. Ochs HD, Slichter SJ, Harker LA, et al. The Wiskott-Aldrich syndrome: studies of lymphocytes, granulocytes, and platelets. Blood 1980;55(2):243–52.

14. Ochs HD, Rosen FS. The Wiskott-Aldrich syndrome. In: Ochs HD, Smith ECI, Puck JM, editors. A molecular and genetic approach. New York: Oxford University Press; 2006. p. 454–69.
15. Vermi W, Blanzuoli L, Kraus MD, et al. The spleen in the Wiskott-Aldrich syndrome: histopathologic abnormalities of the white pulp correlate with the clinical phenotype of the disease. Am J Surg Pathol 1999;23(2):182–91.
16. Meyer-Bahlburg A, Becker-Herman S, Humblet-Baron S, et al. Wiskott-Aldrich syndrome protein deficiency in B cells results in impaired peripheral homeostasis. Blood 2008;112(10):4158–69.
17. Westerberg LS, de la Fuente MA, Wermeling F, et al. WASP confers selective advantage for specific hematopoietic cell populations and serves a unique role in marginal zone B-cell homeostasis and function. Blood 2008;112(10):4139–47.
18. Molina IJ, Sancho J, Terhorst C, et al. T cells of patients with the Wiskott-Aldrich syndrome have a restricted defect in proliferative responses. J Immunol 1993;151(8):4383–90.
19. Trifari S, Sitia G, Aiuti A, et al. Defective Th1 cytokine gene transcription in CD4+ and CD8+ T cells from Wiskott-Aldrich syndrome patients. J Immunol 2006; 177(10):7451–61.
20. Zhang J, Shehabeldin A, da Cruz LA, et al. Antigen receptor-induced activation and cytoskeletal rearrangement are impaired in Wiskott-Aldrich syndrome protein-deficient lymphocytes. J Exp Med 1999;190(9):1329–42.
21. Park JY, Kob M, Prodeus AP, et al. Early deficit of lymphocytes in Wiskott-Aldrich syndrome: possible role of WASP in human lymphocyte maturation. Clin Exp Immunol 2004;136(1):104–10.
22. Orange JS, Ramesh N, Remold-O'Donnell E, et al. Wiskott-Aldrich syndrome protein is required for NK cell cytotoxicity and colocalizes with actin to NK cell-activating immunologic synapses. Proc Natl Acad Sci U S A 2002;99(17):11351–6.
23. Gismondi A, Cifaldi L, Mazza C, et al. Impaired natural and CD16-mediated NK cell cytotoxicity in patients with WAS and XLT: ability of IL-2 to correct NK cell functional defect. Blood 2004;104(2):436–43.
24. Calle Y, Chou HC, Thrasher AJ, et al. Wiskott-Aldrich syndrome protein and the cytoskeletal dynamics of dendritic cells. J Pathol 2004;204(4):460–9.
25. Bouma G, Burns S, Thrasher AJ. Impaired T-cell priming in vivo resulting from dysfunction of WASp-deficient dendritic cells. Blood 2007;110(13):4278–84.
26. Pulecio J, Tagliani E, Scholer A, et al. Expression of Wiskott-Aldrich syndrome protein in dendritic cells regulates synapse formation and activation of naive CD8+ T cells. J Immunol 2008;181(2):1135–42.
27. de Noronha S, Hardy S, Sinclair J, et al. Impaired dendritic-cell homing in vivo in the absence of Wiskott-Aldrich syndrome protein. Blood 2005;105(4):1590–7.
28. Ochs HD, Thrasher AJ. The Wiskott-Aldrich syndrome. J Allergy Clin Immunol 2006;117(4):725–38 [quiz: 739].
29. Dupuis-Girod S, Medioni J, Haddad E, et al. Autoimmunity in Wiskott-Aldrich syndrome: risk factors, clinical features, and outcome in a single-center cohort of 55 patients. Pediatrics 2003;111(5 Pt 1):e622–7.
30. Schurman SH, Candotti F. Autoimmunity in Wiskott-Aldrich syndrome. Curr Opin Rheumatol 2003;15(4):446–53.
31. Strom TS. The thrombocytopenia of WAS: a familial form of ITP? Immunol Res 2009;44(1–3):42–53.
32. Pessach IM, Notarangelo LD. X-linked primary immunodeficiencies as a bridge to better understanding X-chromosome related autoimmunity. J Autoimmun 2009; 33(1):17–24.

33. Humblet-Baron S, Sather B, Anover S, et al. Wiskott-Aldrich syndrome protein is required for regulatory T cell homeostasis. J Clin Invest 2007;117(2):407–18.
34. Maillard MH, Cotta-de-Almeida V, Takeshima F, et al. The Wiskott-Aldrich syndrome protein is required for the function of CD4(+)CD25(+)Foxp3(+) regulatory T cells. J Exp Med 2007;204(2):381–91.
35. Marangoni F, Trifari S, Scaramuzza S, et al. WASP regulates suppressor activity of human and murine CD4(+)CD25(+)FOXP3(+) natural regulatory T cells. J Exp Med 2007;204(2):369–80.
36. Astrakhan A, Ochs HD, Rawlings DJ. Wiskott-Aldrich syndrome protein is required for homeostasis and function of invariant NKT cells. J Immunol 2009; 182(12):7370–80.
37. Locci M, Draghici E, Marangoni F, et al. The Wiskott-Aldrich syndrome protein is required for iNKT cell maturation and function. J Exp Med 2009;206(4):735–42.
38. Tran H, Nourse J, Hall S, et al. Immunodeficiency-associated lymphomas. Blood Rev 2008;22(5):261–81.
39. Ochs HD, Filipovich AH, Veys P, et al. Wiskott-Aldrich syndrome: diagnosis, clinical and laboratory manifestations, and treatment. Biol Blood Marrow Transplant 2009; 15(Suppl 1):84–90.
40. Kanegane H, Nomura K, Miyawaki T, et al. X-linked thrombocytopenia identified by flow cytometric demonstration of defective Wiskott-Aldrich syndrome protein in lymphocytes. Blood 2000;95(3):1110–1.
41. Yamada M, Ariga T, Kawamura M, et al. Determination of carrier status for the Wiskott-Aldrich syndrome by flow cytometric analysis of Wiskott-Aldrich syndrome protein expression in peripheral blood mononuclear cells. J Immunol 2000;165(2):1119–22.
42. Zhu Q, Watanabe C, Liu T, et al. Wiskott-Aldrich syndrome/X-linked thrombocytopenia: WASP gene mutations, protein expression, and phenotype. Blood 1997; 90(7):2680–9.
43. Jin Y, Mazza C, Christie JR, et al. Mutations of the Wiskott-Aldrich syndrome protein (WASP): hotspots, effect on transcription, and translation and phenotype/genotype correlation. Blood 2004;104(13):4010–9.
44. Ramesh N, Anton IM, Hartwig JH, et al. WIP, a protein associated with Wiskott-Aldrich syndrome protein, induces actin polymerization and redistribution in lymphoid cells. Proc Natl Acad Sci U S A 1997;94(26):14671–6.
45. de la Fuente MA, Sasahara Y, Calamito M, et al. WIP is a chaperone for Wiskott-Aldrich syndrome protein (WASP). Proc Natl Acad Sci U S A 2007;104(3): 926–31.
46. Davis BR, Candotti F. Revertant somatic mosaicism in the Wiskott-Aldrich syndrome. Immunol Res 2009;44(1–3):127–31.
47. Bach FH, Albertini RJ, Joo P, et al. Bone-marrow transplantation in a patient with the Wiskott-Aldrich syndrome. Lancet 1968;2(7583):1364–6.
48. Bortin MM, Bach FH, van Bekkum DW, et al. 25th anniversary of the first successful allogeneic bone marrow transplants. Bone Marrow Transplant 1994;14(2): 211–2.
49. Parkman R, Rappeport J, Geha R, et al. Complete correction of the Wiskott-Aldrich syndrome by allogeneic bone-marrow transplantation. N Engl J Med 1978;298(17):921–7.
50. Kapoor N, Kirkpatrick D, Blaese RM, et al. Reconstitution of normal megakaryocytopoiesis and immunologic functions in Wiskott-Aldrich syndrome by marrow transplantation following myeloablation and immunosuppression with busulfan and cyclophosphamide. Blood 1981;57(4):692–6.

51. Ochs HD, Lum LG, Johnson FL, et al. Bone marrow transplantation in the Wiskott-Aldrich syndrome. Complete hematological and immunological reconstitution. Transplantation 1982;34(5):284–8.

52. Reisner Y, Kapoor N, Kirkpatrick D, et al. Transplantation for severe combined immunodeficiency with HLA-A, B, D, DR incompatible parental marrow cells fractionated by soybean agglutinin and sheep red blood cells. Blood 1983;61(2):341–8.

53. Reinherz EL, Geha R, Rappeport JM, et al. Reconstitution after transplantation with T-lymphocyte-depleted HLA haplotype-mismatched bone marrow for severe combined immunodeficiency. Proc Natl Acad Sci U S A 1982;79(19):6047–51.

54. Brochstein JA, Gillio AP, Ruggiero M, et al. Marrow transplantation from human leukocyte antigen-identical or haploidentical donors for correction of Wiskott-Aldrich syndrome.
J Pediatr 1991;119(6):907–12.

55. Antoine C, Muller S, Cant A, et al. Long-term survival and transplantation of haemopoietic stem cells for immunodeficiencies: report of the European experience 1968-99. Lancet 2003;361(9357):553–60.

56. Filipovich AH, Stone JV, Tomany SC, et al. Impact of donor type on outcome of bone marrow transplantation for Wiskott-Aldrich syndrome: collaborative study of the International Bone Marrow Transplant Registry and the National Marrow Donor Program. Blood 2001;97(6):1598–603.

57. Kobayashi R, Ariga T, Nonoyama S, et al. Outcome in patients with Wiskott-Aldrich syndrome following stem cell transplantation: an analysis of 57 patients in Japan. Br J Haematol 2006;135(3):362–6.

58. Pai S-Y, De Martiis D, Forino C, et al. Stem cell transplantation for the Wiskott-Aldrich syndrome: a single-center experience confirms efficacy of matched unrelated donor transplantation. Bone Marrow Transplant 2006;38(10):671–9.

59. Buckley RH. Molecular defects in human severe combined immunodeficiency and approaches to immune reconstitution. Annu Rev Immunol 2004;22:625–55.

60. Conley ME, Saragoussi D, Notarangelo L, et al. An international study examining therapeutic options used in treatment of Wiskott-Aldrich syndrome. Clin Immunol 2003;109(3):272–7.

61. Knutsen AP, Wall DA. Umbilical cord blood transplantation in severe T-cell immunodeficiency disorders: two-year experience. J Clin Immunol 2000;20(6):466–76.

62. Thomson BG, Robertson KA, Gowan D, et al. Analysis of engraftment, graft-versus-host disease, and immune recovery following unrelated donor cord blood transplantation. Blood 2000;96(8):2703–11.

63. Al-Ghonaium A. Stem cell transplantation for primary immunodeficiencies: King Faisal Specialist Hospital experience from 1993 to 2006. Bone Marrow Transplant 2008;42(Suppl 1):S53–6.

64. Ayas M, Al-Seraihi A, A-Jefri A, et al. Unrelated cord blood transplantation in pediatric patients: a report from Saudi Arabia. Bone Marrow Transplant 2009. [Epub ahead of print].

65. Bhattacharya A, Slatter MA, Chapman CE, et al. Single centre experience of umbilical cord stem cell transplantation for primary immunodeficiency. Bone Marrow Transplant 2005;36(4):295–9.

66. Díaz de Heredia C, Ortega JJ, Diaz MA, et al. Unrelated cord blood transplantation for severe combined immunodeficiency and other primary immunodeficiencies. Bone Marrow Transplant 2008;41(7):627–33.

67. Jaing T-H, Tsai BY, Chen SH, et al. Early transplantation of unrelated cord blood in a two-month-old infant with Wiskott-Aldrich syndrome. Pediatr Transplant 2007; 11(5):557–9.
68. Kaneko M, Watanabe T, Watanabe H, et al. Successful unrelated cord blood transplantation in an infant with Wiskott-Aldrich syndrome following recurrent cytomegalovirus disease. Int J Hematol 2003;78(5):457–60.
69. Knutsen AP, Steffen M, Wassmer K, et al. Umbilical cord blood transplantation in Wiskott Aldrich syndrome. J Pediatr 2003;142(5):519–23.
70. Lee PP, Chen TX, Jiang LP, et al. Clinical and molecular characteristics of 35 Chinese children with Wiskott-Aldrich syndrome. J Clin Immunol 2009;29(4): 490–500.
71. Tsuji Y, Imai K, Kajiwara M, et al. Hematopoietic stem cell transplantation for 30 patients with primary immunodeficiency diseases: 20 years experience of a single team. Bone Marrow Transplant 2006;37(5):469–77.
72. Inagaki J, Park YD, Kishimoto T, et al. Successful unmanipulated haploidentical bone marrow transplantation from an HLA 2-locus-mismatched mother for Wiskott-Aldrich syndrome after unrelated cord blood stem cell transplantation. J Pediatr Hematol Oncol 2005;27(4):229–31.
73. Slatter MA, Bhattacharya A, Flood TJ, et al. Use of two unrelated umbilical cord stem cell units in stem cell transplantation for Wiskott-Aldrich syndrome. Pediatr Blood Cancer 2006;47(3):332–4.
74. Filipovich A. Hematopoietic cell transplantation for correction of primary immunodeficiencies. Bone Marrow Transplant 2008;42(Suppl 1):S49–52.
75. Friedrich W, Schuetz C, Schulz A, et al. Results and long-term outcome in 39 patients with Wiskott-Aldrich syndrome transplanted from HLA-matched and -mismatched donors. Immunol Res 2009;44(1–3):18–24.
76. Ozsahin H, Cavazzana-Calvo M, Notarangelo LD, et al. Long-term outcome following hematopoietic stem cell transplantation in Wiskott-Aldrich syndrome: collaborative study of the European Society for Immunodeficiencies and the European Group for Blood and Marrow Transplantation. Blood 2008;11(1):238–44.
77. Yamaguchi K, Ariga T, Yamada M, et al. Mixed chimera status of 12 patients with Wiskott-Aldrich syndrome (WAS) after hematopoietic stem cell transplantation: evaluation by flow cytometric analysis of intracellular WAS protein expression. Blood 2002;100(4):1208–14.
78. Kang HJ, Shin HY, Ko SH, et al. Unrelated bone marrow transplantation with a reduced toxicity myeloablative conditioning regimen in Wiskott-Aldrich syndrome. J Korean Med Sci 2008;23(1):146–8.
79. Rao K, et al. Improved survival after unrelated donor bone marrow transplantation in children with primary immunodeficiency using a reduced-intensity conditioning regimen. Blood 2005;105(2):879–85.
80. De Saint-Basile G, Schlegel N, Caniglia M, et al. X-linked thrombocytopenia and Wiskott-Aldrich syndrome: similar regional assignment but distinct X-inactivation pattern in carriers. Ann Hematol 1991;63(2):107–10.
81. Stewart DM, Candotti F, Nelson DL. The phenomenon of spontaneous genetic reversions in the Wiskott-Aldrich syndrome: a report of the workshop of the ESID Genetics Working Party at the XIIth Meeting of the European Society for Immunodeficiencies (ESID). Budapest, Hungary October 4-7, 2006. J Clin Immunol 2007;27(6):634–9.
82. Mullen CA, Anderson KD, Blaese RM. Splenectomy and/or bone marrow transplantation in the management of the Wiskott-Aldrich syndrome: long-term follow-up of 62 cases. Blood 1993;82(10):2961–6.

83. Bosticardo M, Marangoni F, Aiuti A, et al. Recent advances in understanding the pathophysiology of Wiskott-Aldrich syndrome. Blood 2009;113(25):6288–95.

84. Small TN, Friedrich W, O'Reilly RJ. Hematopoietic cell transplantation for immunodeficiency diseases. In: Appelbaum FR, Forman SJ, Negrin RS, et al, editors. Thomas' hematopoietic cell transplantation. Wiley-Blackwell; 2009. p. 1105–24.

85. Albert MH, Bittner TC, Nonoyama S, et al. X-linked thrombocytopenia (XLT) due to WAS mutations: clinical characteristics, long-term outcome, and treatment options. Blood 2010. [Epub ahead of print].

# Hematopoietic Stem Cell Transplantation for Chronic Granulomatous Disease

Reinhard A. Seger, MD

**KEYWORDS**

- Immunodeficiency • High-risk patient • RIC regimen
- In vivo T-depletion

Chronic granulomatous disease (CGD) is a primary immunodeficiency disease (PID) that affects 1:200,000 live births and is caused by the lack of 1 of 5 subunits of the superoxide-producing nicotinamide adenine dinucleotide phosphate (NADPH) oxidase of neutrophils, macrophages, and eosinophils. In healthy subjects, superoxide is converted into microbicidal reactive oxygen species and indirectly liberates and activates complementary microbicidal azurophil granule proteases[1] and microbicidal neutrophil extracellular traps.[2] NADPH oxidase deficiency thus renders the patient susceptible to recurrent, life-threatening infections by certain bacteria and fungi (eg, by *Aspergillus* sp). The resulting infectious foci stimulate granuloma formation, partly through release and persistence of chemoattractants that require oxygen metabolites for their degradation.[3–5] Chronic granulomatous inflammation can compromise vital organs and account for additional morbidity.

Most patients are diagnosed with CGD in early childhood. Current prophylaxis with co-trimoxazole, itraconazole, and additional interferon gamma is efficient but imperfect often due to resistant fungal infections. Recent progress toward new antibiotic and antifungal therapies allows survival of patients into their 30s.[6,7] Adolescent and adult CGDs, however, are increasingly characterized by hyperinflammatory noninfectious complications, such as granulomatous lung disease and inflammatory bowel disease, requiring immunosuppressive therapy.[8] Allogeneic hematopoietic stem cell transplantation (HSCT) is currently the only curative treatment for CGD and can be offered to selected patients. Improved outcome with supportive care and high clinical variability in the disease course, however, make selection of eligible patients for HSCT difficult. This article addresses recent progress in HSCT for CGD, delineates present limitations, and points to future developments.

Division of Immunology/Hematology/BMT, University Children's Hospital, Steinwiesstrasse 75, Zürich 8032, Switzerland
*E-mail address:* Reinhard.Seger@kispi.uzh.ch

Immunol Allergy Clin N Am 30 (2010) 195–208
doi:10.1016/j.iac.2010.01.003      immunology.theclinics.com

## INDICATIONS FOR HSCT

CGD is a slowly progressing, chronic immunodeficiency with acute exacerbations and accumulating organ sequelae over the years. The median survival of patients on co-trimoxazole/itraconazole long-term therapy in the recently analyzed CGD cohort in United Kingdom is 30 years, with an approximate annual mortality of 2% per year.[7] The transition of pediatric care into adult care is a difficult step because of nonavailability of trained PID specialists in internal medicine in many regions, intermittent compliance to medication, accumulating organ (eg, lung) dysfunction, and increased transplant-related mortality (TRM) (eg, by graft-versus-host disease [GvHD] and organ toxicity) if late HSCT is performed. In addition, there is an almost complete lack of quality-of-life data for adult CGD. This uncertain long-term perspective and the difficulty to define a risk score based on immunologic or genetic laboratory parameters[9] have led the Working Party Inborn Errors of the European Blood and Marrow Transplantation (EBMT) group toward a pragmatic clinical approach to indications for HSCT.

Treatment differs in standard-risk patients (without infection or inflammatory disease at HSCT) and in high-risk patients (with active infection/inflammation) (**Table 1**). Standard risk includes nonavailability of specialist care or noncompliance with antibiotic prophylaxis, both known to increase mortality. Other standard risks are 1 or more life-threatening infections in the past and/or severe granulomatous disease with progressive organ dysfunction (eg, lung restriction), because both predict long-term progression of the disease. Standard-risk patients generally have a good outcome after HSCT if a human leukocyte antigen (HLA)–matched donor (sibling or unrelated) is found.[10]

High-risk patients have ongoing therapy-refractory infection (eg, aspergillosis) or steroid-dependent granulomatous disease (eg, colitis). They are candidates for difficult salvage HSCTs, with HLA-matched donors using special reduced-intensity conditioning (RIC) regimens[10] (see later discussion) in well-experienced PID HSCT centers only. If possible, salvage HSCTs should be delayed using the whole spectrum of modern antifungal therapy or modern immunosuppression first, until high-risk patients have clinically improved or are in remission. In such situations, extensive surgeries such as pneumonectomies or total colectomies should be withheld in favor of HSCT.

To avoid high-risk situations later on, several PID HSCT centers recommend HSCT to all young children with CGD if an HLA-genoidentical sibling is available. This seems justified in view of the low TRM of approximately 5% using a sibling donor, but cannot yet be recommended, if only a matched unrelated donor (MUD) is available (actual TRM of approximately 15%, see later discussion).

**Table 1**
**HLA-matched HSCT for CGD: indications**

| Standard-Risk Patient (Absence of Infection/Inflammation) | High-Risk Patient (Active Infection/Inflammation) |
|---|---|
| One life-threatening infection in the past | Ongoing therapy-refractory infection (eg, aspergillosis) |
| Severe granulomatous disease with progressive organ dysfunction (eg, lung restriction) | Steroid-dependent granulomatous disease (eg, colitis) |
| Nonavailability of specialist care | |
| Noncompliance with antibiotic prophylaxis | |

If HSCT is indicated for standard risk, but no HLA-matched donor is available, several families have successfully opted for in vitro fertilization (IVF) followed by preimplantation genetic diagnosis (PGD), providing an HLA-genoidentical savior baby.[11,12] This ethically difficult indication is discussed later.

If salvage HSCT is indicated, but no HLA-matched donor is available, there are highly experimental alternatives that can be tempted. These include mismatched donor HSCT (only anecdotal experience in CGD) and somatic gene therapy (not curative to date).[13]

## PRETRANSPLANTATION EVALUATION

Detailed pretransplantation evaluation is of critical importance, especially in high-risk and older CGD patients. The extent of tissue damage and organ dysfunction caused by chronic inflammation needs to be carefully evaluated. The presence and nature of infected/inflammatory foci have to be identified using combined positron emission tomography–computed tomography (PET-CT)[14] to guide biopsies of all metabolically active areas for histologic and microbiologic evaluation. Active inflammation (eg, colitis) has to be attended appropriately by immunosuppressive agents. Active infections should be treated adequately using antimicrobials with intracellular action[6] before and during HSCT. Isolated abscesses with difficult access (eg, in brain or liver) need not be drained before HSCT if antimicrobial coverage can be ascertained. Unmatched granulocyte transfusions should be avoided pretransplant because of sensitization of the recipient to multiple HLA and human neutrophil alloantigens.

Patients with X-linked CGD should also be evaluated for a contiguous gene syndrome, manifesting as McLeod red blood cell (RBC) syndrome, retinitis pigmentosa, and Duchenne muscular dystrophy. Patients with McLeod syndrome lack Kx and Kell antigens to which they may have become sensitized by previous transfusions. They need special blood cell support to be organized before HSCT as described in the next section.

## PREPARATIVE REGIMENS
### Myeloablative Conditioning

The number of reports on successful HSCTs in patients with CGD has increased during the past 2 decades. HSCTs were first performed using HLA-genoidentical sibling donors,[10] followed recently by the inclusion of MUDs.[15,16] Initially, RIC regimens resulted in autologous recovery and suggested the necessity for high-dose myeloablative conditioning, a protocol successfully used by members of the Working Party Inborn Errors of the EBMT group (Fig. 1). It relies on a total dose (TD) of busulphan of 16 mg/kg (preferably given intravenously [IV]) with dose adjusted to blood levels and on cyclophosphamide, 200 mg/kg TD. Full marrow is given, and an efficient prophylaxis of GvHD and graft rejection is provided by in vivo T-cell depletion, for example, by alemtuzumab (Campath-1H) at 0.5 to 1 mg/kg TD for MUDs and 0.3 mg/kg TD for matched sibling donors (MSDs). Although myeloablative regimens are successful in obtaining full donor chimerism with long-term survival, the increased risk of worsening infection/inflammation accompanied by severe GvHD and regimen-related toxicity must not be ignored, especially in high-risk and older CGD patients.

### Submyeloablative Conditioning

Ten pediatric/adult patients with CGD were treated at the National Institutes of Health with RIC and T-cell depleted HLA-genoidentical allografts.[17] RIC consisted of

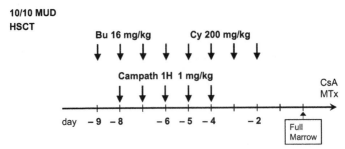

**Fig. 1.** MUD HSCT for CGD: myeloablative protocol. Bu, busulphan; Cy, cyclophosphamide; CsA, cyclosporin A; MTX, methotrexate.

fludarabine, 125 mg/m$^2$ TD, and cyclophosphamide, 120 mg/kg TD, with antithymocyte globulin (ATG), 40 mg/kg TD, and cyclosporin A (CsA) for GvHD prophylaxis. With this regimen, 2 patients rejected the graft and 3 additional patients developed GvHD more than grade II after rescue donor lymphocyte infusions (DLIs). Three of the adult patients died because of serious infections and GvHD, so that this minimal intensive conditioning procedure and the T-cell depletion of HLA-identical grafts were suspended. Japanese transplant centers have later modified this approach by adding a submyeloablative dose of total body irradiation (TBI) of 2 to 4 Gy to the chemotherapy regimen and by using T-cell–replete marrow. This Japanese RIC approach can be an alternative option for high-risk CGD but still comprises a significant risk of graft rejection and GvHD, particularly if DLIs have to be used to ensure engraftment.[18]

Subsequently, some patients with CGD were treated with a European RIC protocol relying on fludarabine, 150 mg/m$^2$ TD, and melphalan, 140 mg/m$^2$ TD. Enthusiasm for this RIC regimen, which had been successful in many other PIDs, diminished as cases of low engraftment level (4%)[19] and late graft failure[20,21] were observed in CGD.

Recently, a modified Slavin RIC regimen has been introduced by the author's group in patients with CGD older than 5 years[22] and has shown to be successful in a pilot cohort of MSD and MUD donors (see later discussion). This protocol relies on fludarabine, 180 mg/m$^2$ TD, IV busulphan of 50% to 60% of the myeloablative TD, achieved by targeting a total area under the curve (AUC) of 50,000 to 60,000 ng·hr/μL, and in vivo T-cell depletion by Campath-1H, as well as GvHD/rejection prophylaxis by CsA and mycophenolate mofetil. This regimen ensures full donor chimerism, avoids severe acute GvHD (>grade II), and graft failure. It is now evaluated by the Working Party Inborn Errors of the EBMT group, also including younger children known to metabolize busulphan at an accelerated rate. Main prerequisite for the protocol is the ability to provide immediate busulphan dose adjustment according to kinetics (AUC) (**Fig. 2**).

## PROPHYLAXIS OF GVHD AND REJECTION

In a CGD transplantation model in noninfected NADPH oxidase–deficient mice, exuberant inflammation was noted after allogeneic HSCT.[23] Irradiated gp91phox −/− mice conditioned with cyclophosphamide were given donor bone marrow in the presence of allogeneic T cells. They subsequently showed marked infiltration of the lungs with inflammatory cells in comparison to normal mice, accompanied by increased bronchoalveolar lavage fluid levels of the chemoattractants monocyte chemoattractant protein 1 and macrophage inflammatory protein (MIP) 1α. In addition, impaired clearance of recombinant mouse MIP-1β, injected IV, was observed in the NADPH

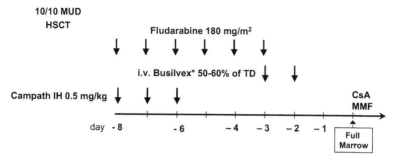

**Fig. 2.** MUD HSCT for CGD: Zürich-RIC protocol. AUC, area under the curve; MMF, mycophenolate mofetil; TD, total dose.

oxidase–deficient mice, likely explaining the enhanced pulmonary influx of inflammatory cells after HSCT. Cultured monocytes/macrophages from gp91phox −/− mice produced 3-fold more tumor necrosis factor (TNF) α than normal mice. In analogy, the increased risk for GvHD in patients with CGD may be because of preexisting inflammation or infection resulting in elevated TNF-α levels. Indeed, a higher incidence of severe GvHD (grade III–IV) was found in patients who had preexisting overt infections and/or active inflammatory conditions, as opposed to standard patients.[10]

Because RIC procedures revealed an increased rejection rate in patients with CGD even in MSD transplants, a balanced in vivo T-cell depletion, depleting host and donor T cells, is now applied in preparative regimens. Polyclonal ATG and monoclonal anti-CD52 antibodies (Campath-1H) are used for depleting not only T cells but also monocyte-derived dendritic cells that express CD52 abundantly.[24] This mitigates presentation of host-derived antigens to donor T cells in the inflammatory peritransplantation environment, limiting GvHD and a severe engraftment syndrome that may result in white lung, occasionally observed in CGD (**Fig. 3**). In vivo T-cell depletion can also avoid late graft failure, but may predispose to CMV reactivation, thus requiring

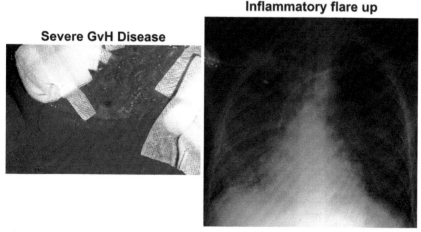

**Fig. 3.** CGD: severe acute complications after HSCT.

careful monitoring for 6 to 9 months posttransplant and preemptive antiviral therapy, if needed.

## CLINICAL RESULTS
### MSD HSCT

Recent MSD transplants for CGD performed in European transplant centers are summarized in **Table 2**. In a historic European series of 27 patients with CGD (1985–2000),[10] 21 received busulphan-based (16 mg/kg TD) myeloablation and full MSD grafts. There was full engraftment in 20 patients and graft failure in none. Severe GvHD (grades III–IV) was observed in 4 patients with severe pretransplant infection or inflammation (eg, aspergillosis or overt colitis). In standard patients, there were only 2 cases of mild grade II GvHD. Three high-risk patients of the cohort died, 1 on day 9 after transplant from disseminated aspergillosis and multiorgan failure, 1 on day 90 from GvHD grade IV and severe engraftment syndrome, and 1 on day 73 from accidental tracheostomy bleeding. Eighteen of the 21 patients (86%) were cured of CGD, had more than or equal to 90% circulating donor myeloid cells, and cleared pre-existing infections and chronic inflammatory lesions. Combined PET-CT showed rapid disappearance of active infections (aspergillosis) and active inflammatory lesions (colitis) within 2 months (**Fig. 4**A, B). Even children with severe lung restriction profited from the transplantation, slowly normalizing decreased oxygen saturation, reversing clubbing of fingers and toes, and manifesting a growth spurt (**Fig. 4**C, D).[10] Similarly, impressive catch-up growth was also seen in transplanted patients with colitis, in whom steroids could be withdrawn.[16] These encouraging results were repeated in 3 recent single-center series, 2 using a myeloablative conditioning[15,16] and 1 a RIC protocol for high-risk patients,[22] with an overall mortality of 1 of 16 (6%) only and no severe GvHD (see **Table 2**).

### MUD HSCT

Recently, 2 reports on successful MUD HSCT using myeloablative conditioning were published.[15,16] The data are summarized in **Table 3**, with additional preliminary data from an ongoing pilot study using RIC.[22,25]

**Table 2**
**Recent MSD transplants for CGD in Europe**

| CGD-Cohort | Patient No | Acute GvHD (Grade) | Graft Failure | Full Engraftment | Mortality | Conditioning |
|---|---|---|---|---|---|---|
| New Castle[16] | 9 | 3/9 (II) | 0/9 | 6/9 (3/9 partial) | 0/9 | Bu 100% Cy 200 |
| Ulm[15] | 3 | 1/3 (II) | 0/3 | 3/3 | 1/3[a] | |
| Zürich[25] | 4 | 0/4 | 0/4 | 4/4 | 0/4 | Bu 50%–60% Flu 180 ATG-F |
| Total | 16 | 4/16 (II) (=25%) | 0/16 | 13/16 (=81%) | 1/16 (=6%) | |
| Europe (historic)[10] | 21 | 6/21 (II–IV) (=28%) | 0/21 | 20/21 (=95%) | 3/21 (=14%) | Bu-based myeloablation |

*Abbreviations:* ATG-F, antithymocyte globulin-Fresenius; Bu, busulphan; Cy, cyclophosphamide; Flu, fludarabine.
[a] Systemic BK viremia.

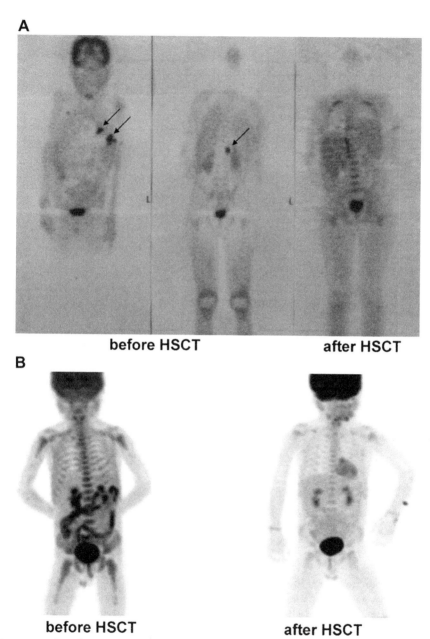

**Fig. 4.** Benefits of HSCT for CGD. (*A*) Recovery from refractory aspergillosis. (*B*) Remission of steroid-dependent colitis. (C) Recovery from chronic lung inflammation. (*D*) Catch-up growth. (*A*) and (*B*) show PET-CT scans. DLCO, carbon monoxide diffusing capacity; FVC, forced vital capacity. (*A, C, D*) (*Data from* Seger RA, Gungor T, Belohradsky BH, et al. Treatment of chronic granulomatous disease with myeloablative conditioning and an unmodified hemopoietic allograft: a survey of the European experience, 1985–2000. Blood 2002;100:4344–50.)

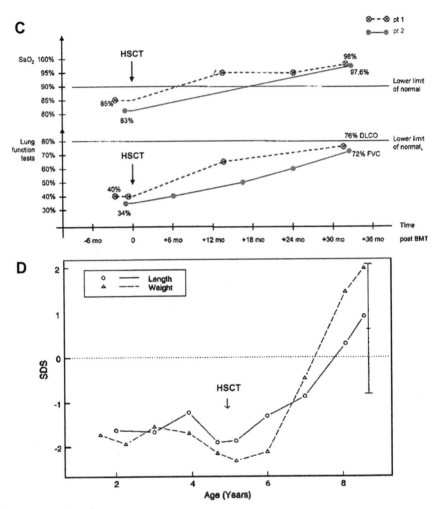

**Fig. 4.** (*continued*)

The overall clinical outcome is similar to MSD HSCT, with a similar rate of engraftment and no severe GvHD. TRM, however, is 10% higher using MUD (16%). Four of 25 patients died, 1 on day 1 from disseminated aspergillosis, 1 on day 532 from the consequences of chronic GvHD after a retransplant, and 2 from acute respiratory distress syndrome (days +28 and +187). In the latter 2 patients, ATG had been used for in vivo T-cell depletion, which may have not resulted in sufficient immunosuppression. The clinical results of RIC for MUD high-risk CGD transplantation were comparable to those of myeloablative conditioning.

### Cord Blood HSCT

There are 4 cases of successful cord blood transplantation for CGD in the literature, using only 4 of 6 or 5 of 6 MUDs and RIC.[26–28] In all cases, engraftment was finally achieved but in 2 patients only after retransplantation. Unrelated cord blood transplantation can thus be a promising alternative strategy in patients with CGD who lack an HLA-identical donor. Clearly, more experience is needed before an optimal preparative regimen (myeloablative conditioning or RIC) can be recommended.

**Table 3**
**Recent MUD transplants for CGD in Europe**

| CGD-Cohort | Patient No | Acute GvHD (Grade) | Graft Failure | Full Engraftment | Mortality | Conditioning |
|---|---|---|---|---|---|---|
| New Castle[16] | 10 | 3/9 (II) | 1/9 (1 retransplant) | 7/9 (1/9 partial) | 1/10[a] | Bu, Cy, Campath-1H (7/10) |
| Ulm[15] | 9 | 3/9 (II) | 2/9 (1 retransplant) | 7/9 | 2/9[b,c] | Bu-based (6/9) |
| Zürich[25] | 6 | 1/6 (II) | 0/6 | 6/6 | 1/6[b] | Bu 50%–60% |
| | | | | | | Flu 180 |
| | | | | | | Campath 0.5 (5/6) |
| Total MUD | 25 | 7/24 (II) (=29%) | 3/24 (=12%) | 20/24 (=83%) | 4/25 (=16%) | |
| Total MSD (see **Table 2**) | 16 | 4/16 (II) (=25%) | 0/16 | 13/16 (=81%) | 1/16 (=6%) | |

[a] Disseminated *Aspergillus nidulans*.
[b] Acute respiratory distress syndrome.
[c] Complication of chronic GvHD.

### Mismatched Donor HSCT

Very few mismatched donor HSCTs have been performed in CGD up to date, mainly in Japan, so that conclusions are not yet possible.[21,29] Haploidentical HSCTs are considered highly risky in infected patients with CGD because of graft failure and delayed immune reconstitution. Their number may increase in the future if gene therapy does not keep up to its promises.

## SPECIAL AREAS IN HSCT
### HSCT with Savior Sibling

HSCT after IVF and combined female sexing and HLA matching offer a therapeutic option for patients with X-linked PID, such as X-CGD, who need HSCT but lack an HLA-identical donor. PGD combined with HLA typing for providing an HLA-identical HSC donor has been accompanied by considerable controversy, and there is no consensus yet as to its authorization. Several criteria must be met to proceed with this strategy[11]: (1) eligible diseases must be severe and benefited by HSCT, (2) only diseases with slow progression are suitable because a minimum of 10 months is required for 1 IVF and PGD cycle with HLA typing followed by the period of gestation, (3) maternal age should be less than 38 years for a sufficient number of retrievable oocytes, and (4) psychological counseling is mandatory to avoid potential instrumentation of the savior child. Parents also have to be informed that birth rates per PGD cycle are low (15% for all published cases). Up to date, there are only 3 reported cases of successful HSCT by an HLA-genoidentical savior sibling in CGD.[11,12]

### HSCT for X-CGD with McLeod Syndrome

X-CGD may rarely be due to a large deletion of the X-chromosomes, including the adjacent *XK* gene. This is associated with the McLeod red cell phenotype, defined by the absence of the Kx protein and by reduced expression of the Kell blood group antigens. Transfusion of RBCs from healthy donors leads to sensitization to Kx in these patients and may induce severe hemolytic transfusion reactions. Suitable blood donors with McLeod phenotype are extremely rare.

Several successful HSCTs in patients with X-CGD/McLeod syndrome have been reported,[30–33] including 1 previously sensitized patient.[33] The following precautions are recommended for such HSCTs: (1) administration of erythropoietin pretransplant, (2) cryopreservation of Kx-negative patient's RBCs, (3) depletion of patient's B cells by anti-CD20, (4) complete myeloablation and immune ablation to avoid mixed chimerism with persistence of Kx- and Kell-sensitized host B and T cells (eg, by TBI 12 Gy TD, fludarabine, 160 mg/m$^2$ TD, and rabbit ATG, 10 mg/kg TD),[33] (5) RBC depletion of Kx-positive transplants, (6) transfusion of Kell-negative packed RBC posttransplant, and (7) DLI for alloimmune hemolysis posttransplant.[32]

### Organ Transplantation After HSCT

Organ transplantation before or after HSCT has been exceptionally reported in CGD. The main indication for renal transplantation in CGD was end-stage renal failure after multiple courses of amphotericin and for liver transplantation it was chronic hepatic GvHD. If stem cell and organ donors are identical, the need for long-term immunosuppression is eliminated by tolerance. When the donors are different, graft rejection may occur infrequently, suggesting that alloimmunity is less robust after HSCT.[34] To avoid allogeneic rejections from passenger lymphocytes in a liver graft, portal vein and hepatic artery were flushed with ablative anti-CD3 antibodies.[35] To date, 4 successful living donor kidney transplants[34,36] and 1 successful living donor liver transplant[35] are reported. Sequential stem cell and organ transplantation requires a multidisciplinary approach before, during, and after transplantation, which has led to success in numerous cases after HSCT for different disease entities.

## FUTURE DIRECTIONS

There is an urgent need for studies to develop better guidelines, especially as to those patients with CGD most likely to benefit from HSCT.[37] Will it be possible in the future to base the indication for or against HSCT in an individual patient on his genotypic, biochemical, or immunologic susceptibility profile for severe infections/inflammatory conditions, as well as on his past clinical course? What is the quality of life of adults with CGD without transplantation in the current era as compared with a multicenter retrospective review of HSCT outcomes done for CGD since 2000?

Mortality and morbidity of HSCT can be reduced by using a less-toxic conditioning regimen compared with conventional myeloablative conditioning. For clinical cure, 10% of stable donor chimerism in the myeloid compartment should be sufficient, provided the corresponding threshold chimerism of X-CGD carriers can be extrapolated.[38] As shown earlier, a modified Slavin conditioning regimen is currently the most promising RIC scheme. The modifications include the necessity to measure IV busulphan levels real time with immediate dose adjustment and the administration of prolonged immunosuppression by in vivo T-cell depletion (by ATG or Campath-1H), together with mycophenolate.[22] This RIC regimen will now be further tested in children younger than 5 years with high-risk CGD who do not tolerate myeloablation. Because of the increased busulphan metabolism in this young age group, higher percentages of the total myeloablative busulphan dose may be needed for engraftment (eg, 60%–70% instead of 50%–60% TD in patients older than 5 years).

Antibody-based minimal-intensity conditioning is now being tested on other patients with PID and may reduce toxicity and late effects even further, especially in patients with preexisting organ dysfunction and in patients younger than 1 year in whom chemotherapy conditioning is poorly tolerated. A novel anti-CD45 antibody–based minimal-intensity conditioning regimen has allowed curative donor stem cell engraftment without nonhemopoietic toxicity in a cohort of patients with PID.[39] Further studies are needed to establish whether this approach can be extended to patients without underlying T-cell defects, including CGD.

## SUMMARY

Despite important advances in supportive therapy, CGD remains a lethal disease, nowadays at an adult age. The only curative approach is allogeneic stem cell transplantation. Clinical outcome is now excellent for MSD (with approximately 5% TRM) and good for MUD (approximately 15% TRM). More patients would be treated by transplantation, provided the inflammatory complications triggered by heavy conditioning and preexisting infection could be prevented in CGD, a proinflammatory disease by its own. RIC combined with moderate in vivo depletion of inflammatory cells is worth pursuing, taking care to preserve some donor T cells needed for engraftment. RIC HSCT has already proved to be a promising treatment modality for older and more fragile patients with CGD with intractable infection or inflammation and is now further tested in smaller children. Ideally, however, infections ought to be under control before starting conditioning.

The decision for or against transplantation should be made early in life when HSCT is best supported and when there are still few disease sequelae. HSCT may be most useful in those patients suffering from recurrent serious infections despite correct antimicrobial prophylaxis or severe steroid-dependent inflammatory complications having a well-matched stem cell or cord blood donor. Uncomplicated CGD, however, is currently only considered an indication for HSCT if an HLA-genoidentical sibling donor is available.

## ACKNOWLEDGMENTS

I am grateful to all transplanted patients affected by CGD who participated in the research efforts that enable this article.

My thanks go to Andrew Cant, Paul Veys, and Tayfun Guengoer for helpful discussions and to Janine Reichenbach for manuscript review.

## REFERENCES

1. Reeves EP, Lu H, Jacobs HL, et al. Killing activity of neutrophils is mediated through activation of proteases by K+ flux. Nature 2002;416:291–7.
2. Fuchs TA, Abed U, Goosmann C, et al. Novel cell death program leads to neutrophil extracellular traps. J Cell Biol 2007;176:231–41.
3. Clark RA, Klebanoff SJ. Chemotactic factor inactivation by the myeloperoxidase-hydrogen peroxide-halide system. J Clin Invest 1979;64:913–20.
4. Hamasaki T, Sakano T, Kobayashi M, et al. Leukotriene B4 metabolism in neutrophils of patients with chronic granulomatous disease: phorbol myristate acetate decreases endogenous leukotriene B4 via NADPH oxidase-dependent mechanism. Eur J Clin Invest 1989;19:404–11.
5. Lekstrom-Himes JA, Kuhns DB, Alvord WG, et al. Inhibition of human neutrophil IL-8 production by hydrogen peroxide and dysregulation in chronic granulomatous disease. J Immunol 2005;174:411–7.
6. Seger RA. Modern management of chronic granulomatous disease. Br J Haematol 2008;140:255–66.
7. Jones LB, McGrogan P, Flood TJ, et al. Special article: chronic granulomatous disease in the United Kingdom and Ireland: a comprehensive national patient-based registry. Clin Exp Immunol 2008;152:211–8.
8. Schappi MG, Jaquet V, Belli DC, et al. Hyperinflammation in chronic granulomatous disease and anti-inflammatory role of the phagocyte NADPH oxidase. Semin Immunopathol 2008;30:255–71.
9. Foster CB, Lehrnbecher T, Mol F, et al. Host defense molecule polymorphisms influence the risk for immune-mediated complications in chronic granulomatous disease. J Clin Invest 1998;102:2146–55.
10. Seger RA, Gungor T, Belohradsky BH, et al. Treatment of chronic granulomatous disease with myeloablative conditioning and an unmodified hemopoietic allograft: a survey of the European experience, 1985-2000. Blood 2002;100:4344–50.
11. Reichenbach J, Van de Velde H, De Rycke M, et al. First successful bone marrow transplantation for X-linked chronic granulomatous disease by using preimplantation female gender typing and HLA matching. Pediatrics 2008;122:e778–82.
12. Goussetis E, Konialis CP, Peristeri I, et al. Successful hematopoietic stem cell transplantation in 2 children with X-linked chronic granulomatous disease from their unaffected HLA-identical sibling selected using preimplantation genetic diagnosis combined with HLA typing. Biol Blood Marrow Transplant 2010;16:344–9.
13. Ott MG, Schmidt M, Schwarzwaelder K, et al. Correction of X-linked chronic granulomatous disease by gene therapy, augmented by insertional activation of MDS1-EVI1, PRDM16 or SETBP1. Nat Med 2006;12:401–9.

14. Gungor T, Engel-Bicik I, Eich G, et al. Diagnostic and therapeutic impact of whole body positron emission tomography using fluorine-18-fluoro-2-deoxy-D-glucose in children with chronic granulomatous disease. Arch Dis Child 2001; 85:341–5.

15. Schuetz C, Hoenig M, Gatz S, et al. Hematopoietic stem cell transplantation from matched unrelated donors in chronic granulomatous disease. Immunol Res 2009; 44:35–41.

16. Soncini E, Slatter MA, Jones LB, et al. Unrelated donor and HLA-identical sibling haematopoietic stem cell transplantation cure chronic granulomatous disease with good long-term outcome and growth. Br J Haematol 2009;145:73–83.

17. Horwitz ME, Barrett AJ, Brown MR, et al. Treatment of chronic granulomatous disease with nonmyeloablative conditioning and a T-cell-depleted hematopoietic allograft. N Engl J Med 2001;344:881–8.

18. Hasegawa D, Fukushima M, Hosokawa Y, et al. Successful treatment of chronic granulomatous disease with fludarabine-based reduced-intensity conditioning and unrelated bone marrow transplantation. Int J Hematol 2008;87:88–90.

19. Petrovic A, Dorsey M, Miotke J, et al. Hematopoietic stem cell transplantation for pediatric patients with primary immunodeficiency diseases at All Children's Hospital/University of South Florida. Immunol Res 2009;44:169–78.

20. Nicholson JA, Wynn RF, Carr TF, et al. Sequential reduced- and full-intensity allografting using same donor in a child with chronic granulomatous disease and coexistent, significant comorbidity. Bone Marrow Transplant 2004;34:1009–10.

21. Kikuta A, Ito M, Mochizuki K, et al. Nonmyeloablative stem cell transplantation for nonmalignant diseases in children with severe organ dysfunction. Bone Marrow Transplant 2006;38:665–9.

22. Gungor T, Halter J, Klink A, et al. Successful low toxicity hematopoietic stem cell transplantation for high-risk adult chronic granulomatous disease patients. Transplantation 2005;79:1596–606.

23. Yang S, Panoskaltsis-Mortari A, Shukla M, et al. Exuberant inflammation in nicotinamide adenine dinucleotide phosphate-oxidase-deficient mice after allogeneic marrow transplantation. J Immunol 2002;168:5840–7.

24. Ratzinger G, Reagan JL, Heller G, et al. Differential CD52 expression by distinct myeloid dendritic cell subsets: implications for alemtuzumab activity at the level of antigen presentation in allogeneic graft-host interactions in transplantation. Blood 2003;101:1422–9.

25. Güngör T, Halter J, Stüssi G, et al. Successful busulfan-based reduced intensity conditioning in high-risk pediatric and adult chronic granulomatous disease (CGD) [abstract]. Bone Marrow Transplant 2009;43:S75.

26. Bhattacharya A, Slatter M, Curtis A, et al. Successful umbilical cord blood stem cell transplantation for chronic granulomatous disease. Bone Marrow Transplant 2003;31:403–5.

27. Parikh SH, Szabolcs P, Prasad VK, et al. Correction of chronic granulomatous disease after second unrelated-donor umbilical cord blood transplantation. Pediatr Blood Cancer 2007;49:982–4.

28. Mochizuki K, Kikuta A, Ito M, et al. Successful unrelated cord blood transplantation for chronic granulomatous disease: a case report and review of the literature. Pediatr Transplant 2009;13:384–9.

29. Miki M, Kajiume T, Nakamura K, et al. Successful marrow transplantation with an intensively immunosuppressive conditioning with low toxicity for high-risk chronic granulomatous disease patients. ASH Annual Meeting Abstracts. Blood 2006; 108:5354.

30. Schuetz C, Hoenig M, Schulz A, et al. Successful unrelated bone marrow transplantation in a child with chronic granulomatous disease complicated by pulmonary and cerebral granuloma formation. Eur J Pediatr 2007;166:785–8.

31. Suzuki N, Hatakeyama N, Yamamoto M, et al. Treatment of McLeod phenotype chronic granulomatous disease with reduced-intensity conditioning and unrelated-donor umbilical cord blood transplantation. Int J Hematol 2007;85:70–2.

32. Kordes U, Binder TM, Eiermann TH, et al. Successful donor-lymphocyte infusion for extreme immune-hemolysis following unrelated BMT in a patient with X-linked chronic granulomatous disease and McLeod phenotype. Bone Marrow Transplant 2008;42:219–20.

33. Hoenig M, Flegel WA, Schwarz K, et al. Successful hematopoietic stem-cell transplantation in a patient with chronic granulomatous disease and McLeod phenotype sensitized to Kx and K antigens. Bone Marrow Transplant 2010;45:209–11.

34. Bolanowski A, Mannon RB, Holland SM, et al. Successful renal transplantation in patients with chronic granulomatous disease. Am J Transplant 2006;6:636–9.

35. Yokoyama S, Kasahara M, Fukuda A, et al. Successful living-donor liver transplantation for chronic hepatic graft-versus-host disease after bone marrow transplantation for chronic granulomatous disease. Transplantation 2008;86:367–8.

36. Peces R, Ablanedo P, Seco M. [Amyloidosis associated with chronic granulomatous disease in a patient with a renal transplant and recurrent urinary tract infections]. Nefrologia 2002;22:486–91 [in Spanish].

37. Griffith LM, Cowan MJ, Kohn DB, et al. Allogeneic hematopoietic cell transplantation for primary immune deficiency diseases: current status and critical needs. J Allergy Clin Immunol 2008;122:1087–96.

38. Segal BH, Leto TL, Gallin JI, et al. Genetic, biochemical, and clinical features of chronic granulomatous disease. Medicine 2000;79:170–200.

39. Straathof KC, Rao K, Eyrich M, et al. Haemopoietic stem-cell transplantation with antibody-based minimal-intensity conditioning: a phase 1/2 study. Lancet 2009;374:912–20.

# Hematopoietic Stem Cell Transplantation for Profound T-cell Deficiency (Combined Immunodeficiency)

Chaim M. Roifman, MD, FRCPC, FCACB

**KEYWORDS**

• HSCT • Profound T cell dysfunction • Mutation • Engraftment

## DESCRIPTION OF PROFOUND T-CELL DEFICIENCY/COMBINED IMMUNODEFICIENCY

Typical cases of severe combined immunodeficiency (SCID) present at infancy (most frequently at 6 months of age) with repeated opportunistic infections; failure to thrive; and scarcity of lymphoid tissues, including undetectable lymph nodes and a small dysplastic thymus. The laboratory hallmark in these cases is profound T-cell lymphopenia.

In the past 2 decades, we have witnessed the discovery and characterization of a growing number of patients who present disorders such as SCID with repeated opportunistic infections, but unlike SCID, they have a significant number of circulating T cells.[1–7] Frequently, these patients may present with a prominent skin rash, enlarged lymph nodes, and a normal-size thymus.[7,8] Some of these patients may have a delayed or atypical presentation beyond one year of age or present with lung granulomas or lymphoid malignancy, whereas others may have associated syndromic features. The terms $T^+$ SCID, CID, and leaky SCID have been frequently used to describe this group of inherited immune disorders that shares a profound T-cell dysfunction (PTD) associated with a significant number of circulating autologous T cells (CD3$^+$ cell count >500 cell/μL and frequently increased). This heterogenous group of disorders includes (1) patients who carry genetic aberration that typically present with autologous T cells (**Table 1**), (2) leaky SCID because of hypomorphic mutations in SCID-causing genes (**Table 2**), (3) multiorgan syndromes associated with PTD (**Table 3**), and (4) PTD with a yet unknown genetic defect.

Division of Immunology/Allergy, The Canadian Centre for Primary Immunodeficiency, The Jeffrey Modell Research Laboratory for the Diagnosis of Primary Immunodeficiency, The Hospital for Sick Children, University of Toronto, 555 University Avenue, Toronto, ON, M5G 1X8, Canada
E-mail address: chaim.roifman@sickkids.ca

Immunol Allergy Clin N Am 30 (2010) 209–219
doi:10.1016/j.iac.2010.03.001
0889-8561/10/$ – see front matter © 2010 Elsevier Inc. All rights reserved.
immunology.theclinics.com

The first group includes PTD/CID disorders in which all known mutations are consistently associated with circulating autologous T cells. Zeta-chain–associated protein kinase 70 (Zap-70),[1] CD3$\gamma$,[9] and interleukin (IL)-2R$\alpha$[2] deficiencies, as well as immunodysregulation polyendocrinopathy enteropathy X-linked syndrome (IPEX), are good representatives of this group.[10] In spite of having a large number of circulating T cells, in vitro responses to anti-CD3 or mitogens are frequently depressed. Some features in these patients may aid in the diagnosis. CD8 lymphocytopenia may suggest a mutation in *Zap-70*,[11] whereas the lack of in-vitro response to exogenous IL-2[12] or the reduced expression of CD3[3] may alert to the possibility of IL-2R$\alpha$ or CD3$\gamma$ deficiency, respectively. IPEX should be suspected in patients with severe intractable gastrointestinal (GI) manifestations presenting early in infancy.[10]

The second group of patients consists of PTD/CID caused by mutations that allow for residual activity, resulting in a substantial "leak" of T cell from the thymus. More

**Table 1**
**Distinct genotypes/phenotypes**

|  | Chromosome/Gene | Immunotype | Phenotype |
|---|---|---|---|
| Zap-70 deficiency (OMIM 176947)[a] | 2q12/*ZAP-70* | T$^+$(CD8 low) B$^+$ MR: reduced Ig: low TM: medulary CD8 lymphopenia | Normal-size thymus and normal-size lymph nodes, opportunistic infections, FTT, Omenn syndrome |
| CD25 deficiency (OMIM 606367)[a] | 10p15-p14/*IL-2R$\alpha$* | T$^+$B$^+$ MR: reduced Ig: low TM: lack of Hassall corpuscles | Endocrinopathy, lymphadenopathy, hepatosplenomegaly, opportunistic infections, FTT, multiorgan autoimmunity |
| PNP deficiency (OMIM 164050)[a] | 14q13.1/*PNP* | T$^+$B$^+$, progressive lymphopenia MR: reduced Ig: low | Ataxia, bone marrow failure, opportunistic infections, FTT, autoimmunity |
| DNA ligase 4 deficiency (OMIM 601837)[a] | 13q33-q34/*LIG4* | T$^+$B$^-$ MR: variable Ig: variable | Microcephaly, growth and developmental delay, autoimmunity, pancytopenia, various skin abnormalities, Omenn syndrome |
| MHC class II deficiency (OMIM 600005)[b] | 16p13/*CIITA* | T$^+$(CD4 low) B$^+$ MR: reduced Ig: low | Opportunistic infections, autoimmunity |
| CD40 ligand deficiency (OMIM 300386)[b] | Xq26/*CD40LG* | T$^+$B$^+$ MR: normal Ig: IgM high, IgG low, low-specific antibodies | PJP pneumonia, lymphoma |

*Abbreviations:* FTT, failure to thrive; Ig, immunoglobulin; MHC, major histocompatibility complex; MR, mitogenic response; PJP, pneumocystis jiroveci pneumonia; PNP, purine nucleoside phosphorylase; TM, thymus morphology; *ZAP-70, zeta-chain–associated protein kinase 70.*
   [a] Candidate for HSCT.
   [b] HSCT may be considered if a full-matched related donor is available.

**Table 2**
**Atypical phenotypes caused by hypomorphic mutations in genes associated with SCID**

| | Chromosome/Gene | Mutation | Immunotype | Phenotype |
|---|---|---|---|---|
| γc (OMIM 308380)[a] | Xq13.1/IL2Rγ | C62X, K97X, G114D, C115R, L151P, I153N, R222C, R267X, L271Q, S286X, and others | T+B+ <br> MR: reduced to normal <br> Ig: low to normal | Opportunistic infections <br> Lymph nodes and thymus shadow present |
| JAK3 (OMIM 600173)[a] | 19p13.1/JAK3 | E481G, C759R, R445X, IVS9AS A-G -2, IVS12DS C-T -20 | T+B+ <br> MR: reduced <br> Ig: normal to increased | Opportunistic infections, FTT, chronic diarrhea, autoimmunity |
| CD3ε (OMIM 186830)[a] | 11q23/CD3ε | W59X | T+B+ <br> MR: reduced <br> Ig: low | Susceptibility to recurrent pneumonia and otitis media |
| CD3γ (OMIM 186740)[a] | 11q23/CD3γ | K69X, M1V, IVS2AS G-C -1 | T+B+ <br> MR: reduced <br> Ig: variable | Susceptibility to infections, autoimmunity |
| RAG-1/RAG-2 (OMIM 179615/179616)[a] | 11p13/RAG-1 <br> 11p13/RAG-2 | R396C/H/L, R561C/H, E722K, A444V, plus others R229W, R148X, F206C, C41W, M285R, R229Q | T+B− , oligoclonality <br> MR: reduced <br> Ig: low | Opportunistic infections, granulomata, autoimmunity, Omenn syndrome |
| ARTEMIS (OMIM 605988)[a] | 10p13/DCLRE1C | M1T, H35D | T+B− , oligoclonality <br> MR: reduced <br> Ig: low | Opportunistic infections, thrombocytopenia, anemia, Omenn syndrome |
| ADA (delayed) deficiency (OMIM 102700)[b] | 20q12-q13.11/ADA | Q3X, G74D, R76W, R149Q, L152M, R211C, A215T, T233I, P274L, P297Q, and others | T+B+ <br> MR: reduced <br> Ig: low | Liver and lung disease, neurologic manifestations, skeletal abnormalities, Omenn syndrome |

*Abbreviations:* ADA, adenosine deaminase; Ig, immunoglobulin; MR, mitogenic response.
[a] Candidate for HSCT.
[b] HSCT may be considered if a full–HLA-matched related donor is available.

**Table 3**
Syndromes that may be associated with CI

| | Chromosome/Gene | Immunotype | Phenotype |
|---|---|---|---|
| Cartilage-hair hypoplasia (OMIM 250250)[a] | 9p21-p12/RMRP | T+B+ MR: variable from severe to mild reduction Ig: variable TM: dysplastic | Short stature, metaphyseal dysplasia, hypoplastic hair, possible anemia/neutropenia, malabsorption and/or aganglionic megacolon, non-Hodgkin lymphoma Omenn syndrome and autoimmunity |
| Wiskott-Aldrich syndrome (OMIM 301000)[a] | Xp11.4-p11.21/WAS | T+(CD8 low) B+ MR: variable, mostly normal Ig: IgM low | Thrombocytopenia, small platelets, eczema, susceptibility to infection, nephropathy, autoimmunity, lymphoreticular malignancy |
| Dyskeratosis congenita XL/Hoyeraal-Hreidarsson syndrome (OMIM 305000/300240) Dyskeratosis congenita AD (OMIM 127550) Dyskeratosis congenita AR (OMIM 224230) | Xq28/DKC1 3q26/TERC 5p15.33/TERT 14q12/TINF2 15q14-q15, 5q35.3/NOLA2, NOLA3 | T+(variable) B−(variable) MR: variable Ig: variable | Bone marrow aplasia, pancytopenia, reticular hyperpigmentation of the skin, poor dentition, osteoporosis, dystrophic nails, premalignant leukokeratosis of the mouth mucosa, pulmonary fibrosis, liver fibrosis, possible ataxia, microcephaly, growth/mental retardation |
| Familial intestinal polyatresia (OMIM 243150) | N/A | T+B+ MR: reduced Ig: low TM: dysplastic | Recurrent infections, intraluminal calcifications, intestinal atresia, prematurely born and small for gestational age |

| Disease | Gene/locus | Immune phenotype | Clinical features |
| --- | --- | --- | --- |
| Roifman-Costa syndrome (Roifman syndrome II) (OMIM 300258) | N/A | $T^+B^+$ MR: reduced Ig: low | Short stature, metaphyseal dysplasia, autoimmunity (RA, SLE), recurrent infections |
| Dionisi Vici syndrome (OMIM 234150) 242840) | N/A | $T^+$(low) $B^+$ MR: variable Ig: low TM: dysplastic | Recurrent opportunistic infections, agenesis of the corpus callosum, oculocutaneous hypopigmentation/albinism, cataracts, cleft lip and palate, cardiomyopathy, postnatal growth retardation, microcephaly and profound developmental delay |
| Ataxia-telangiectasia (OMIM 208900) | 11q22-q23/ATM | $T^+B^+$ (low) MR: variable Ig: variable TM: dysplastic | Cerebellar ataxia, telangiectasia, predisposition to cancer |
| Nijmegen breakage syndrome (OMIM 251260) | 8q21/NBS1 | $T^+$ (low) $B^+$ (low) MR: low Ig: low | Microcephaly, growth retardation, predisposition to cancer |

Abbreviations: Ig, immunoglobulin; MR, mitogenic response; RA, rheumatoid arthritis; SLE, systemic lupus erythematosus.
[a] Candidate for HSCT.

deleterious mutations in these genes result in SCID. Some of these patients present with severe erythroderma, eosinophilia, lymphadenopathy, and hepatosplenomegaly, which are the hallmarks of Omenn syndrome (OS). Invariably, such patients have a restricted T-cell repertoire with oligoclonal T-cell expansion. Most of these patients have extremely low to undetectable CD19[+] or CD20[+] B cells, and a molecular diagnosis can be made in more than 50% of these cases (hypomorphic mutations in *recombination activating gene (RAG) 1/RAG-2, ARTEMIS, or DNA ligase 4*).[13–15] In other patients with OS, the number of circulating B cells may be normal or elevated. Mutations in the *RMRP*,[7] $\gamma c$,[16] and *IL-7R$\alpha$*[17] as well as *adenosine deaminase (ADA)*,[18] were identified in some of these cases. Regardless of the genetic defect, patients with OS benefit from effective suppression of T-cell clonal expansion followed by a hematopoietic stem cell transplantation (HSCT).

More difficult to diagnose are cases with hypomorphic mutations in SCID-causing genes but with no OS features. Most frequently, these patients also have a full T-cell repertoire or close to normal representation of all V$\beta$ families.

Typical examples of these cases are patients who carry the R222C mutation in the $\gamma c$ chain. Some of these cases may have normal lymphocyte count and near-normal in vitro mitogenic responses.[4,5]

The third group includes profound immunodeficiency that can also be associated with various multisystem syndromes such as ADA deficiency,[18] cartilage-hair hypoplasia (CHH),[7] or DNA ligase 4.[19] The degree of immunodeficiency in syndromic PTD varies widely from SCID to very mild, barely significant immunodeficiency. This has been clearly shown in CHH.[20] ADA deficiency can also be variable, with some mutations being more commonly associated with a SCID phenotype, whereas others with delayed or partial ADA deficiency.[21]

The degree of PTD/CID[1] has to be carefully assessed before a decision on HSCT can be made. The decision should also take into consideration the effect of nonimmune manifestations on the patients' outcome. For instance, CHH could be an indication for HSCT but not ataxia telangiectasia.

Finally, in the fourth group, there are still many cases with PTD/CID[9] in which the genetic basis of their defect remains unknown. Such patients suffer frequent infections requiring hospitalization as well as severe autoimmune manifestations that can lead to permanent end-organ damage and death. Rarely, a full evolution of the immune system cannot decisively lead to the diagnosis of PTD; in other patients, primary immunodeficiency cannot be easily distinguished from secondary immunodeficiency. In these cases, analysis of thymus histology can be extremely useful. This strategy has been proved safe and beneficial to patients because a decision regarding HSCT can be made early rather than late, thus improving outcome of the procedure.

Two striking examples of this successful strategy have been the identification of an abnormal thymus in patients with CD8 lymphocytopenia.[11] Patients received a successful HSCT, 4 years before the discovery of the genetic aberration in the *Zap-70* gene.[1] In a similar fashion, the patient with IL-2R$\alpha$ deficiency received a successful HSCT several years before a mutation in *CD25* was identified.[2]

Although normal thymus morphology may not exclude the possibility of profound T-cell deficiency,[22] abnormal thymus morphology (ie, lack of Hassall corpuscles and/or loss of thymic architecture) is consistently found only in biopsies or autopsies of infants with primary immunodeficiency.[22]

Because the procedure is safe even in the hands of less-experienced surgeons, benefits seem to outweigh risks in cases in which no other test can substantiate the diagnosis of PTD/CID.

## GUIDELINES FOR DIAGNOSIS AND TREATMENT OF PTD/CID

After excluding secondary causes of immunodeficiency (human immunodeficiency virus, drugs), PTD may be suspected in patients who have 1 or a combination of the following features:

1. A presentation with typical infections (such as pneumocystis pneumonia, cytomegalovirus pneumonitis, oral thrush, and recurrent invasive infections)
2. Atypical presentation with lymphoid malignancy, severe GI manifestations, or granuloma/autoimmunity
3. Decreased or deteriorating function of circulating T cells
4. CD3$^+$ T-cell numbers are usually greater than 500 cells/$\mu$L and frequently increased (OS)
5. Low T-cell receptor excision circles (TRECs) (or CD4RA) and/or restricted diversity of the T-cell repertoire
6. Significant mutation in a gene involved in T-cell function and/or evidence of defective expression/function of the encoded protein
7. Abnormal thymus morphology (dysplastic changes such as lack of Hassall corpuscles and abnormal architecture)
8. Family history of profound T-cell deficiency
9. Signs and symptoms relevant to syndromes, which may be associated with profound T-cell deficiency, such as
   - Short stature—CHH
   - Microcephaly—DNA ligase 4 deficiency.

HSCT can be recommended if (**Fig. 1**)

1. A presentation with typical infections or OS features is supported by in vitro depressed mitogenic responses (<20% of control) or molecular diagnosis and/or a dysplastic thymus
2. Atypical presentation (lymphoma, granuloma/autoimmunity) supported by molecular diagnosis or dysplastic thymus
3. Immunodeficiency is the major feature of the disorder, and HSCT is likely to cure, reduce morbidity, or prolong life.

## CHOICE OF STEM CELL TRANSPLANTATION

Patients with PTD/CID have moderate to large numbers of circulating autologous lymphocytes with variable residual function. These cells may interfere with proper engraftment and may complicate the procedure of HSCT, hence the need for conditioning. Some of these cells maybe of maternal origin, but their numbers seem to be small in most cases.

Survival rates of these patients post-HSCT with no conditioning was traditionally low, suggesting that ablation of recipient hematopoietic system may be necessary. Whether myeloablative regimens are essential in all cases of PTD/CID and in all types of HSCT remains to be carefully studied. Nevertheless, the authors have been using full myeloablative doses of busulfan and cyclophosphamide in all cases with exceptional results.

The optimal donor for these patients remains a relative with an identical HLA typing (related identical donor [RID]). But such donors are found for only a minority of patients.

As an alternative, HSCT from HLA-mismatched related donors (MMRDs) has been commonly attempted[23,24] for SCID as well as PTD/CID. Compiled European experience shows an overall survival of 54%, with even lower rates in cases of OS and

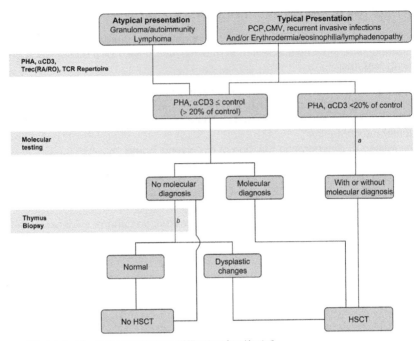

a Molecular testing is important but even in its absence, HSCT can be performed (see text).
b Thymus biopsy can be an important diagnostic tool in these circumstances.

**Fig. 1.** Flowchart for management of PTD.

PTD/CID. Furthermore, careful analysis in a single-center experience demonstrated only 25% to 30% survival rate in cases in which patients received frank haploidentical (half-matched) transplant of MMRD.[25] Further, recent studies have suggested a time-dependent loss of engraftment after MMRD HSCT, including progressive lymphopenia, restricted T-cell repertoire, decreased thymic output, and abnormal humoral immunity.[26]

In 1988, the authors chose to use matched unrelated donor (MUD) HSCT in all cases of PTD/CID. The first patient to receive a MUD HSCT presented with OS and pneumonitis caused by *Pneumocystis jiroveci*. The patient is now 21 years old and healthy while sustaining a robust engraftment and normal cellular as well as humoral immunity.[27] The authors have since transplanted 19 patients with PTD/CID, of which 7 received an RID, whereas 12 received MUD HSCT.[28,29] One patient with RID died of severe lung disease, whereas 1 patient in the MUD group died of graft-versus-host disease (GvHD) (**Table 4**). Patients have been observed for up to 20 years, and immune function was fully evaluated once immunosuppression (GvHD prophylaxis) has been discontinued, usually 1 to 2 years posttransplant. Evaluation included chimerism, complete blood cell count markers, mitogenic responses, TREC copies, assessment of T-cell receptor repertoire, immunoglobulins, and specific antibodies. Immune evaluation was performed at least in part on yearly basis.[27,29]

All patients demonstrated sustained complete T-cell engraftment. All patients had robust T-cell function and normal specific antibodies.

Complications included most commonly acute GvHD. In most cases, GvHD was well managed with additional immunosuppression or a pulse of methylprednisolone.[30] Still, prolonged GvHD was the direct culprit of death in 1 of the patients. Remarkably, the frequency of severe infections has been low. A major complication of HSCT in

**Table 4**
**Outcome of HSCT for PTD/CID**

| Patient | HSCT | Immune Deficiency/ Genetic Defect | Outcome |
|---------|------|-----------------------------------|---------|
| 1 | MUD | γc | AW |
| 2 | MUD | γc | AW |
| 3 | MUD | γc | AW |
| 4 | MUD | Omenn/UK | AW |
| 5 | MUD | UK | AW |
| 6 | MUD | Omenn/UK | AW |
| 7 | MUD | Omenn/UK | AW |
| 8 | MUD | Omenn/UK | AW |
| 9 | MUD | Omenn/*RMRP* | AW |
| 10 | MUD | UK | AW |
| 11 | MUD (cord) | UK | AW |
| 12 | MUD | Omenn/*RMRP* | AW |
| 13 | MUD | UK | Dead, GvHD |
| 14 | RID | Zap-70 | AW |
| 15 | RID | Zap-70 | AW |
| 16 | RID | Omenn | Dead, fatal lung disease |
| 17 | RID | IL-2Rα | AW |
| 18 | RID | Omenn/*RMRP* | AW |
| 19 | RID | UK | AW |
| 20 | RID | CD40L | AW |

*Abbreviations:* AW, alive and well; MUD, matched unrelated donor; RID, related identical donor; UK, unknown.

SCID is life-threatening infections, especially of the lower respiratory tract. Indeed, interstitial pneumonitis is the most frequent cause of death in patients who received MMRD HSCT.[31] In contrast, patients with PTD/CID had on average only 1 major episode of infection while convalescing from RID or MUD HSCT. Yet, 1 patient with OS who presented with severe lung disease eventually died of respiratory failure.

There is no immediate explanation for this excellent outcome of HSCT for PTD/CID. Historically, protocols for MMRD HSCT did not include conditioning regimens, which could jeopardize engraftment. In addition, after conditioning, engraftment is rapid, thus possibly reducing the frequency of infections in these patients. Nevertheless, careful studies on the role of conditioning, especially myeloablative conditioning, should be conducted in the future. It is possible that in some genotypes, RID can be accepted by the recipient with little or no conditioning. Until such studies become instructive, the protocols in current use seem to provide excellent, although not perfect, outcome in patients with PTD/CID.

**REFERENCES**

1. Arpaia E, Shahar M, Dadi H, et al. Defective T cell receptor signaling and CD8+ thymic selection in humans lacking Zap-70 kinase. Cell 1994;76:947–58.

2. Sharfe N, Dadi HK, Shahar M, et al. Human immune disorder arising from muta-tion of the α chain of the interleukin-2 receptor. Proc Natl Acad Sci U S A 1997;94: 3168–71.
3. Alarcon B, Regueiro JR, Arnaiz-Villena A, et al. Familial defect in the surface of expression of the T-cell receptor CD3 complex. N Engl J Med 1988;319: 1203–8.
4. Sharfe N, Shahar M, Roifman CM. An interleukin-2 receptor γ chain mutation with normal thymus morphology. J Clin Invest 1997;100:3036–43.
5. Somech R, Roifman CM. Mutation analysis should be performed to rule out γc deficiency in children with functional severe combined immune deficiency despite apparently normal immunologic tests. J Pediatr 2005;147:555–7.
6. Zhang J, Quintal L, Atkinson A, et al. Novel RAG1 mutation in a case of severe combined immunodeficiency. Pediatrics 2005;116:e445–9.
7. Roifman CM, Gu Y, Cohen A. Mutations in the RNA component of Rnase MRP cause Omenn syndrome. J Allergy Clin Immunol 2006;117:897–903.
8. Notarangelo LD, Giliani S, Mazza C, et al. Of genes and phenotypes: the immu-nological and molecular spectrum of combined immune deficiency: defects of the gamma(c)-JAK3 signaling pathway as a model. Immunol Rev 2000;178: 39–48.
9. Timon M, Arnaiz-Villena A, RodroAguez-Gallego C, et al. Selective disbalances of peripheral blood T lymphocyte subsets in human CD3 gamma deficiency. Eur J Immunol 1993;23:1440.
10. Bennet CL, Christie J, Ramsdell F, et al. The immune dysregulation, polyendoc-rinopathy, enteropathy, X-linked syndrome (IPEX) is caused by mutations of FOXP3. Nat Genet 2001;27(1):20–1.
11. Roifman CM, Hummel DB, Martinez-Valdez H, et al. Depletion of CD8+ cells in human thymic medulla results in selective immune deficiency. J Exp Med 1989; 170(6):2177–82.
12. Roifman CM. Human IL-2 receptor alpha chain deficiency. Pediatr Res 2000; 48(1):6–11.
13. Villa A, Santagata S, Bozzi F, et al. Partial V(D)J recombination activity leads to Omenn syndrome. Cell 1998;93:885–96.
14. Or Ege M, Ma Y, Manfras B, et al. Omenn syndrome due to ARTEMIS mutations. Blood 2005;105(11):4179–86.
15. Grunebaum E, Bates A, Roifman CM. Omenn syndrome is associated with muta-tions in DNA ligase IV. J Allergy Clin Immunol 2008;122(6):1219–20.
16. Shibata F, Toma T, Wada T, et al. Skin infiltration of CD56(bright) CD16(-) natural killer cells in a case of X-SCID with Omenn syndrome like manifestations. Eur J Haematol 2007;79:81–5.
17. Giliani S, Bonfim C, de Saint Basile G, et al. Omenn syndrome in an infant with IL7RA gene mutation. J Pediatr 2006;148:272–4.
18. Roifman CM, Zhang J, Atkinson A, et al. Adenosine deaminase deficiency can present with features of Omenn syndrome. J Allergy Clin Immunol 2008;121(4): 1056–8.
19. van der Burg M, van Veelen LR, Verkaik NS, et al. A new type of radiosensitive T-B-NK+ severe combined immunodeficiency caused by a LIG4 mutation. J Clin Invest 2006;116:137–45.
20. Makitie O, Kaitila I. Cartilage-hair-hypoplasia—clinical manifestations in 108 Finnish patients. Eur J Pediatr 1993;152:211–7.
21. Santisteban I, Arredondo-Vega FX, Kelly S, et al. Three new adenosine deami-nase mutations that define a splicing enhancer and cause severe and partial

phenotypes: implications for evolution of a CpG hotspot and expression of a transduced ADA cDNA. Hum Mol Genet 1995;4:2081–7.

22. Roifman CM. Studies of patients' thymi aid in the discovery and characterization of immunodeficiency in humans. Immunol Rev 2005;203:143–55.

23. Antoine C, Muller S, Cant A, et al. Long-term survival and transplantation of hae-mopoietic stem cells for immunodeficiencies: report of the European experience 1968–99. Lancet 2003;33:1089–95.

24. Haddad E, Landais P, Friedrich W, et al. Long-term immune reconstitution and outcome after HLA-nonidentical T-cell depleted bone marrow transplantation for severe combined immunodeficiency: a European retrospective study of 116 patients. Blood 1998;91:3646–53.

25. Caillat-Zucman S, Le Deist F, Haddad E, et al. Impact of HLA matching on outcome of hematopoietic stem cell transplantation in children with inherited diseases: a single-centre comparative analysis of genoidentical, haploidentical or unrelated donors. Bone Marrow Transplant 2004;33:1089–95.

26. Ball LM, Lankester AC, Bredius RG, et al. Graft dysfunction and delayed immune reconstitution following haploidentical peripheral blood hematopoietic stem cell transplantation. Bone Marrow Transplant 2005;35(Suppl 1):S35–8.

27. Dalal I, Reid B, Doyle J, et al. Matched unrelated bone marrow transplantation for combined immunodeficiency. Bone Marrow Transplant 2000;25:613–21.

28. Guggenheim R, Somech R, Grunebaum E, et al. Bone marrow transplantation for cartilage-hair-hypoplasia. Bone Marrow Transplant 2006;38:751–6.

29. Nahum A, Reid B, Grunebaum E, et al. Matched unrelated bone marrow trans-plant for Omenn syndrome. Immunol Res 2009;44(1–3):25–34.

30. Somech R, Kavadas FD, Atkinson A, et al. High-dose methylprednisolone is effective in the management of acute graft-versus-host disease in severe combined immune deficiency. J Allergy Clin Immunol 2008;122(6):1215–6.

31. Grunebaum E, Mazzolari E, Porta F, et al. Bone marrow transplantation for severe combined immune deficiency. JAMA 2006;295(5):508–18.

# Bone Marrow Transplantation and Alternatives for Adenosine Deaminase Deficiency

H. Bobby Gaspar, MRCP(UK), PhD, MRCPCH

**KEYWORDS**

- Adenosine deaminase • Severe combined immunodeficiency
- Stem cell gene therapy • Enzyme replacement therapy

Severe combined immunodeficiency (SCID) arises from several different genetic defects. The majority of these abnormalities relate to factors that are specific to the immune system and which lead to lymphoid-specific lineage development abnormalities. In contrast to this is adenosine deaminase (ADA)-deficient SCID, which is thought to comprise approximately 10% to 15% of all cases of SCID.[1] ADA is an enzyme involved in the purine salvage pathway that is required for the recycling of adenosine (Ado) and deoxyadenosine (dAdo) after DNA breakdown, and is expressed in all tissues of the body. The absence of ADA enzyme activity through naturally inherited mutations in the ADA gene leads to the buildup of intracellular and extracellular substrates, all of which have adverse effects on the functions of different cell types. The clinical effects of ADA deficiency are manifest in different organ systems, but most dramatically so in the immune system where it leads to severe lymphopenia with abnormal development of T, B, and natural killer (NK) cells.

ADA deficiency, like other forms of SCID, is invariably fatal in the first year of life and requires early intervention. Hematopoietic stem cell transplantation (HSCT) remains the mainstay of treatment but, unlike for other forms of SCID, 2 other treatment options are available, namely enzyme replacement therapy (ERT) with PEG-ADA and autologous hematopoietic stem cell gene therapy (GT). These different options have coexisted for at least the last decade, and in the case of ERT and HSCT for at least 2 decades. In this article the author reviews the available data on treatment by these

Conflict of interest statement: The author is an occasional consultant to Enzon.
Centre for Immunodeficiency, Molecular Immunology Unit, UCL Institute of Child Health, 30 Guilford Street, London WC1N 1EH, UK
*E-mail address:* h.gaspar@ich.ucl.ac.uk

Immunol Allergy Clin N Am 30 (2010) 221–236
doi:10.1016/j.iac.2010.01.002
0889-8561/10/$ – see front matter © 2010 Elsevier Inc. All rights reserved.

different options, and offers an overview on when each of the different treatment options should be used.

## BIOCHEMICAL BASIS OF ADA-SCID

ADA (EC3.5.4.4) is an enzyme of the purine salvage pathway, expressed at different levels in all tissues of the body, with the highest levels detected in the thymus. ADA catalyzes the conversion of deoxyadenosine (dAdo) and adenosine (Ado) to deoxyinosine and inosine, respectively (**Fig. 1**).[1] In the absence of ADA activity, dAdo accumulates in extracellular compartments and within cells, where it is converted by the enzyme deoxycytidine kinase (dCydK) to deoxyadenosine triphosphate (dATP). The buildup of both dATP and dAdo has deleterious effects on lymphocyte development and function, and is the major cause of the immunologic defects. dATP inhibits ribonucleotide reductase, an enzyme that participates in DNA replication and repair,[2] induces apoptosis in immature thymocytes,[3] and interferes with terminal deoxynucleotidyl transferase (TdT) activity, thus limiting V(D)J recombination and antigen receptor diversity.[4] dAdo accumulation inactivates the enzyme S-adenosylhomocysteine hydrolase (SAHH),[5] resulting in inhibition of transmethylation reactions necessary for effective lymphocyte activation. Elevated levels of Ado, acting through cell surface G protein coupled receptors, may contribute to immune dysfunction[6,7] and pulmonary inflammation associated with ADA deficiency.[8] However, the profound

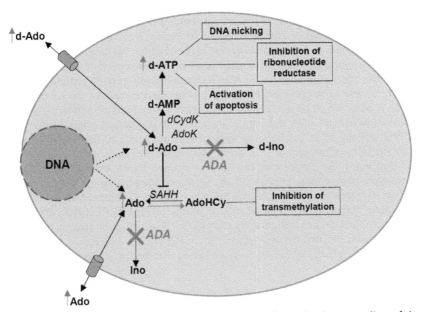

**Fig. 1.** Pathogenesis of ADA deficiency. The breakdown of DNA leads to recycling of deoxyadenosine and adenosine. In the absence of ADA, deoxyadenosine is converted to deoxyadenosine triphosphate and adenosine is converted to S-adenosylhomocysteine, both of whose substrates adversely affect several intracellular mechanisms. ADA, adenosine deaminase; ADCY, adenylyl cyclase; Ado, adenosine; AdoHCy, S-adenosylhomocysteine; AdoK, adenosine kinase; d-Ado, 2-deoxyadenosine; d-AMP, deoxyadenosine monophosphate; d-ATP, deoxyadenosine triphosphate; dCydK, deoxycytidine kinase; d-Ino, deoxyinosine; Ino, inosine; SAHH, S-adenosylhomocysteine hydrolase.

and relatively selective lymphopenia of ADA deficiency may be best explained by the expression pattern of ADA, which is highest in the thymus as a result of high lymphocyte turnover,[9,10] and also by increased expression of dCydK in lymphocytes, which increases dATP accumulation from dAdo in immune cells more than in other tissues.[11]

The expression of ADA throughout the body does, however, lead to several significant nonimmunologic defects. ADA-SCID patients have been noted to have costochondral abnormalities and skeletal dysplasias,[12] neurologic deficits involving motor function,[13] cognitive and behavioral defects,[14,15] bilateral sensorineural deafness,[16] and hepatic dysfunction.[17] Several of these abnormalities are present despite correction of immunologic abnormalities after bone marrow transplantation,[14] thus highlighting the systemic nature of the disease. Nonimmunologic deficits are also found in ADA-deficient mice, which exhibit hepatocyte degeneration, pulmonary and intestinal defects,[18–20] and neurologic abnormalities,[21] with dATP and dAdo accumulation and SAHH inhibition in affected tissues.

## PRINCIPLES FOR THE MANAGEMENT OF ADA DEFICIENCY

The pathogenesis of ADA-SCID arises from the accumulation of toxic metabolites in intra- and extracellular compartments. The nucleosides Ado and dAdo are transported to the plasma once the catalytic activity of dCydK is saturated, whereas dATP is trapped inside the cells. In principle, any form of treatment that aids the clearance of Ado and dAdo from the plasma will shift the dynamic equilibrium of metabolites from within cells and then achieve detoxification, ultimately promoting immune recovery. Thus delivery of sufficient ADA enzyme, whether exogenously (eg, ERT) or packaged within cells (allogeneic stem cell transplant or GT), is the goal for correction of the disease phenotype.

## HEMATOPOIETIC CELL TRANSPLANTATION

Hematopoietic cell transplantation (HCT), if available, has been considered the mainstay of treatment for ADA-SCID. HCT is the most readily available treatment for most transplant centers and, if successful, offers permanent correction of the disease. The protocols for the use of HSCT in ADA-SCID and the outcome following these procedures have, however, not been formally reported and with the availability of different treatment options, there remains some uncertainty on when to use transplant and what protocols to use for conditioning. Until very recently, the only data available have come from large follow-up studies on SCID in general where the numbers of ADA-SCID transplants were in the minority. The largest series to be found is a report from the European SCETIDE database, which documents outcome on 475 SCID transplants, 51 of whom were ADA-deficient patients.[22] The 3-year survival data demonstrate an 81% survival for ADA-SCID patients undergoing an HLA-matched donor transplant and 29% survival for those patients undergoing parental mismatched transplants, with no outcome data on the 4 patients undergoing a matched unrelated procedure. In another study of 94 SCID patients transplanted at 2 separate centers, 6 patients were reported and showed 4 matched related donor transplants (3 survivors) and 2 unrelated donor transplants (1 survivor).[23] These data do not effectively represent the use of unrelated donor transplants and importantly do not address several issues, including whether conditioning is necessary for the various different treatment options and also the degree of immune reconstitution and chimerism following the different transplant procedures. There is also a perception from clinicians that ADA-SCID patients are more difficult to transplant than other SCID patients, and that these patients are more vulnerable to conditioning or infection perhaps as a result of the underlying metabolic defect.

For these reasons, a multicenter retrospective analysis on outcome of transplant for ADA-SCID was initiated, involving European and North American centers. Interim analyses have been presented at European Group for Blood and Marrow Transplantation meetings and were summarized in a recent review article.[24] The major outcomes reported were that matched sibling (n = 31) and matched donor transplants (n = 8) were highly successful, with 3-year survival figures of 87% and 88%, respectively. Matched unrelated donor transplant (n = 11) survival figures were 67%, but much poorer figures were obtained for mismatched related donor transplants (n = 30) (from haploidentical parental donors) where survival was only 43%. The survival following mismatched unrelated transplants was similarly only 29% (n = 7). The reasons for the divergent survival figures are difficult to dissect out, but the major determining factors appear to be HLA disparity and the use of conditioning. The availability of a fully matched related donor does allow the infusion of the donor graft without the need for any prior cytoreductive conditioning regime. The majority of transplants in the matched sibling and matched family donor setting were undertaken without any conditioning and therefore avoided the chemotherapy-related toxicities to which these patients are anecdotally vulnerable. For other donor options for which the outcome figures are less good, the use of conditioning may have played a major factor. It may be argued that given the minimal residual immunity present in ADA-SCID patients, it is possible to perform all transplants without the use of conditioning even in the unrelated and haploidentical setting. However, the data available do not support this. Of 4 unrelated donor transplants performed without conditioning, 2 did not engraft effectively. Data are also available for ADA-SCID haploidentical transplants performed without conditioning.[25] Of 19 procedures performed at a single North American institution, 14 survived (73%) the procedure but only 7 patients were successfully engrafted (disease-free survival 37%) with the remainder rejecting the unconditioned transplant. Together, these data suggest that unconditioned transplants can only be successfully undertaken with fully matched sibling and family donors, but there is a need for cytoreductive conditioning for all other donor types.

Other determining factors were also examined. The perceived susceptibility of ADA-SCID to conditioning has led to the suggestion that patients may benefit from reduced intensity procedures but interestingly, there was no difference between patients undergoing reduced intensity conditioning (n = 8, survival = 50%) and those undergoing fully myeloablative conditioning (n = 38, survival = 50%). The use of PEG-ADA prior to transplant has been argued as both a positive and negative risk factor. Some have argued that its use before transplant may stabilize children and therefore improve transplant outcome. In contrast, others argue that its use may blunt the survival advantage to ADA-containing donor cells. In this study at least, neither argument prevails as no difference in survival was found between those who received PEG-ADA before transplant and those who did not.

One important outcome noted was the quality of immune recovery. The data available suggest that the majority of patients who survive transplant normalize absolute lymphocyte and T-cell counts. Impressively, 92% of patients were able to discontinue immunoglobulin replacement therapy, including 24 of 26 patients undergoing unconditioned sibling donor procedures, suggesting that immune recovery is relatively complete in the majority of surviving patients. Similarly, patients are well detoxified after transplant with marked reduction of dATP levels to a mean of approximately 100 mmol/L which, although not normal, represents approximately 1 log reduction from levels at diagnosis.

No data were available on the degree of donor chimerism. The author's own experience suggests that following unconditioned procedures, the majority of patients only show donor T-cell engraftment, which may be complete or mixed. However, there is little donor cell engraftment in myeloid or B-cell lineages. Other data from animal experiments suggest that in murine neonatal transplants in ADA-deficient mice, engraftment of ADA-replete cells in nonlymphoid organs such as liver or in myeloid cells can lead to cross-correction and development of endogenous T cells.[26] The inference from these different observations is that what is important is not necessarily engraftment of donor cells in any specific lineage but, as alluded to earlier, the delivery of sufficient ADA enzyme in an engrafting cellular source that allows effective systemic detoxification, thereby promoting T- and B-cell development.

An important question for this disease has been the effect of transplantation on the other manifestations of ADA-SCID. Follow-up of transplanted patients demonstrates that despite effective immune recovery and stable detoxification, the majority of patients show cognitive deficits, with a mean IQ score 2 standard deviations below the population normal range, and also show hyperactivity and attention deficit patterns of behavioral disorders.[15] Patients also show a high incidence of audiological problems, with a typical pattern of high-frequency sensorineural hearing loss. For both types of defect, it was not possible to make any correlation with the type of transplant or the conditioning regime, or the degree of chimerism, metabolic detoxification, or immune recovery. The only variable to influence outcome was the level of dATP at the time of diagnosis, which showed a negative correlation with the IQ level, suggesting that greater metabolic derangement at diagnosis led to poorer IQ.[14] This result would suggest that a certain amount of damage may be present at birth that is irreversible, despite immune and metabolic reconstitution, which may relate in part to in utero damage to the developing fetus and may argue for earlier therapeutic intervention.

These data provide some useful guidance on the use of transplant following different donor options. The results from matched sibling donor and matched related donors are extremely good and similar to those seen for other forms of SCID. The ability to undertake these procedures without chemotherapy and thereby avoid long- and short-term chemotherapy-related toxicities makes this a very attractive option, as does the documented quality of cellular and humoral immune reconstitution. By contrast, mismatched transplants especially from parental donors are poorly tolerated and have poor survival figures. These transplants are also unsuccessful without any conditioning, with a high rate of rejection, and therefore it would be advisable to avoid such procedures altogether given that other treatment options such as ERT and GT are available. Matched unrelated donor (MUD) transplants were still poorly represented in this series, with only 11 fully matched procedures undertaken and an overall survival rate of 67%; it is difficult to make any firm recommendation on the basis of such small numbers (see also the later general discussion alongside the use of other treatment options). The ability to avoid nonimmunologic complications is not influenced by the type of transplant or the degree of conditioning, and it is presently not possible to recommend any specific measures.

## ENZYME REPLACEMENT THERAPY

Enzyme replacement therapy (ERT) with PEG-ADA (Adagen, Enzon Inc; obtained outside USA through Orphan Europe) for the treatment of ADA deficiency has been available for almost 20 years and has been designated an orphan drug. The use of PEG-ADA provides another treatment modality for ADA-SCID, but unlike HSCT or

GT it is not a curative therapy but requires regular intramuscular administration. Nevertheless, the effectiveness of PEG-ADA in correcting metabolic and immunologic parameters and, more importantly, in promoting clinical well-being in patients makes it an important option in the care of patients.

PEG-ADA is a compound in which the bovine form of ADA is covalently conjugated to polyethylene glycol (PEG). Pegylation confers several therapeutically beneficial properties to ADA through alteration of its physical and chemical properties, mainly due to an increase in molecular weight.[27,28] The circulating life of the compound is prolonged from minutes to days as clearance from the circulation is inhibited. Pegylation also reduces the immunogenicity of a protein, which again helps to extend its circulating life.[27]

PEG-ADA is administered by once- or twice-weekly intramuscular injections, and results in high levels of ADA activity in the plasma. Of importance is that PEG-ADA cannot cross the cellular membrane and therefore exerts its effect through extracellular ADA activity. High ADA activity in the plasma eliminates Ado and dAdo and, because of the equilibrium maintained between the intra- and extracellular compartments, this results in the movement of Ado and dAdo into the extracellular compartment where further deamination occurs. By drawing adenosine from the cell, this then reduces intracellular accumulation of dATP and its consequent toxic effects.

Since the first patients were treated, the dosing regime has evolved and it is now advised that children should start at a dose of 60 U/kg/wk with biweekly injections until metabolic correction is established (between 1 and 3 months). Once patients show clinical improvement and biochemical stabilization, they can be maintained on a dose of 30 U/kg/wk in a single weekly injection.[29,30] It is important when monitoring patients to assess their immune function as well as metabolic parameters, and this should be taken into account when considering altering the dose of PEG-ADA. Erythrocyte dATP levels can also be measured and used to guide treatment. Initial trough plasma ADA levels (before injection) should be maintained at 50 to 150 μmol/h/ml (normal range <0.4 μmol/h/ml), which equates to approximately 4 to 10 times the normal erythrocyte ADA activity and is required for initial rapid detoxification. Once a maintenance dose of 30 U/kg/wk is established, trough plasma ADA levels can be maintained at 25 to 60 μmol/h/ml. Erythrocyte deoxyadenosine nucleotide levels decrease significantly, and are maintained at levels below those observed after HSCT and SAHH activity is normalized. It is recommended that trough plasma ADA activity levels are monitored every 1 to 2 weeks during the first 2 to 3 months of treatment, twice a month until 9 months of treatment, and then monthly until 18 to 24 months on PEG-ADA. Once patients are established on an effective maintenance dose then plasma ADA levels can be measured every 2 to 4 months unless there is a change in clinical status.

## IMMUNE RECONSTITUTION ON PEG-ADA

Immune reconstitution following treatment with PEG-ADA has not as yet been reported in a formal manner, and the data cited here are taken from retrospective and single-center studies. The impression from these different studies is that immune recovery is variable, the reasons for which may be associated with the underlying clinical condition of the child, the age at which treatment is started, and the level of residual thymic activity at the time of PEG-ADA initiation. Up to 20% of patients receiving therapy appear to show no response.[1,30] In the majority of cases, however, full immune recovery is seen in the short term but is followed by waning T-cell numbers.[31] In terms of humoral immunity, continued immunoglobulin replacement is required in up to 50% of those treated[25] with long term PEG-ADA. What is not clearly documented, however, since most attention has been directed toward immune recovery, is that following PEG-ADA initiation, there is rapid detoxification of dATP levels and this is temporally associated with an increased clinical well-being in patients who start to feed and gain weight. Over time, despite patients having suboptimal immune function, similarly there is well-maintained clinical well-being, with freedom from infection and good growth parameters.

Immune recovery is evidenced initially by an increase in B-cell numbers within a few weeks of starting treatment, and is followed by an increase in T-cell count that may take several months to occur. Symptoms of immune dysregulation such as hemolytic anemia and immune thrombocytopenia can be seen during this period, and may be related to dysregulated cellular and humoral recovery. Recovery of T cells following initiation of PEG-ADA is variable. Again a formal description of T-cell recovery in large numbers of patients is not available but the author's practice has seen 2 major patterns of T-cell recovery. There are patients who show T-cell recovery with regeneration of CD4 and CD8 populations and the development of some naïve T-cell precursors. Over time, these individuals run levels of T cells that are below the normal range for age and are significantly T-lymphopenic. The other pattern seen and which appears to be most common is patients who show T-cell recovery but this being composed almost entirely of memory T cells. In these individuals, despite maintaining high levels of ADA activity and effective detoxification, very little CD4 T-cell and especially naïve CD4 T-cell output is seen. It is most probable that in these patients there has been, either in utero or in the early neonatal stage, significant damage to the thymus as a result of high levels of circulating toxic metabolites. The capacity for these individuals to generate naïve T cells through ERT appears to be severely limited, and such individuals are protected by the development of more mature T-cell populations.

Data on long-term outcome in patients with ADA deficiency treated with PEG-ADA has been published by several groups.[25,32,33] Chan and colleagues[33] published a retrospective review of 9 patients treated in North America with follow-up data from 1995 to 2002. The patients were mostly typical ADA-SCID patients with early presentation (one late-onset patient) who had received PEG-ADA for 5 to 15 years. Their clinical course over this time was good, with little in the way of recurrent or severe infections, although any immune reconstitution associated with treatment declined over time. The majority of children also received other forms of treatment including HSCT and GT. Absolute lymphocyte counts (ALC) remained below the normal range despite improving from baseline. ALC peaked between 1 and 3 years on PEG-ADA at 250 to 1480 cells/mm$^3$, but fell after 5 to 12 years of therapy to 12 to 500 cells/mm$^3$. Proliferative responses normalized in some patients after an average of 4 months of treatment before declining over time. Immunoglobulin production was difficult to assess as patients received supplemental immunoglobulin. Again it was postulated that limited thymic reserve or age-related decline in thymic function may have given rise to the decrease in T-cell numbers over time.

Malacarne and colleagues[32] explored thymic output and immune reconstitution in 5 patients (ages 5–9 years) with ADA-SCID treated with PEG-ADA for 5 to 8 years. B-cell and T-cell numbers again increased 5 to 14 months following initiation of treatment, but remained low in comparison with normal controls. Patient responses to phytohemagglutinin (mitogen) stimulation increased but were variable even within the same patient. Four of the 5 patients developed specific antibodies after immunization with tetanus and showed an increase in serum immunoglobulin levels. Normal T-cell development and thymic output were measured through T-cell receptor excision circles (TRECS), and these proved to be consistently low compared with healthy age-matched controls, again suggesting a compromise in thymic function. B-cell repertoire was examined and found to be restricted, but it is not clear if this relates to an intrinsic B-cell problem or is secondary to defects in the T-cell compartment. Patients remained clinically well on long-term therapy with PEG-ADA.

A European survey of patients receiving PEG-ADA therapy was undertaken in 2005 and preliminary data were published in 2007.[25] Data gathered from 42 patients based in several European centers showed that PEG-ADA was started in the first 6 months of life in over half of the patients (n = 27). Two-thirds of patients received PEG-ADA only and the remainder progressed to HSCT or GT. Four reported deaths were infection related (cytomegalovirus viremia, respiratory syncytial virus infection, encephalitis, and pneumonitis) and were unlikely to be related to PEG-ADA. As previously reported, immune recovery was variable, with T-lymphocyte numbers below the normal range after 1 year of treatment (mean CD3+ count: 460 cells/mm$^3$). Immunoglobulin levels improved to the extent that 40% of patients received immunoglobulin replacement after 1 year. Overall survival in this cohort was 85% for children who received PEG-ADA alone (n = 26). Survival for those who went on to receive HSCT was 70% and 100% for those progressing to GT.

At present the long-term consequences of PEG-ADA therapy are unknown, but it is clear that immune recovery especially in the T-cell compartment is below normal levels and in some patients runs at levels that are of concern with regard to opportunistic infection. The reasons for this have not been determined, but reduced thymic function either at the onset of therapy or over the course of therapy may play an important role. The majority of patients have remained clinically well without experiencing major infective problems, but several case reports suggest that in certain patients ongoing low T-cell numbers has led to significant problems. One boy developed Hodgkin lymphoma after 13 years of treatment,[31] another developed Burkitt lymphoma again after 13 years of treatment,[34] and another child developed Epstein-Barr virus–positive malignant brain lymphoma after 10 years of treatment.[35] It is likely that such lymphoproliferative disease arises due to reduced immune surveillance. Further data gathering is necessary to determine overall outcome of patients on long term therapy.

The effects of PEG-ADA on the metabolic disturbances and immune reconstitution seen in ADA deficiency have been well described, but its effect on systemic manifestations of disease in not clear. In several major centers, children with ADA deficiency proceed to HSCT when an appropriate donor becomes available and PEG-ADA treatment is discontinued, and therefore long-term systemic outcome data are lacking. In those patients who have remained on long-term ERT, there are no formal data on the outcome of systemic pathology. The cognitive and behavioral abnormalities and sensorineural deafness described in ADA-deficient patients are certainly not affected by metabolic correction and persist after transplantation; these are now well documented, but no such data exist for patients on PEG-ADA. This lack of data perhaps is because no individual center has a sufficiently large cohort on long-term ERT to perform such a study and because such studies, especially on behavioral function, are difficult to perform across several different countries and continents.

The development of specific IgG antibody to bovine peptide epitopes of PEG-ADA has been reported by several groups, and often coincides with an improvement in humoral immunity.[25,30,36,37] There are no reports of antibody formation to PEG itself; it can be detected by enzyme-linked immunosorbent assay in up to 80% of patients on long-term PEG-ADA therapy but is clinically insignificant in most. Neutralizing antibodies to PEG-ADA that directly inhibit catalytic activity and accelerate clearance from plasma have been identified in 9 patients.[36,37] Seven of these patients were able to either continue ERT after dosage adjustment, or they underwent successful HSCT. However, loss of efficacy contributed to death in 4 patients, including 3 who also developed refractory hemolytic anemia.

The development and use of PEG-ADA has provided an important alternative option for treatment of patients with ADA deficiency. The rapid metabolic detoxification afforded by high-level enzyme replacement allows clinical stabilization of patients and provides longer-term treatment options when no suitable donor is available. The long-term immune recovery on PEG-ADA appears to be suboptimal, although clinical well-being is maintained in the majority of patients. However, PEG-ADA is not readily available in all countries, which together with its high cost may limit its applicability to all patients.

## GENE THERAPY FOR ADA-DEFICIENT SCID

ADA-SCID has long been seen as an attractive target for hematopoietic cell GT. Indeed the very first clinical trials of GT for any genetic disease were performed on patients with ADA-SCID in the early 1990s. The reasons for its emergence as an ideal target disorder for GT include (1) its monogenic nature; (2) its role as a "housekeeping" enzyme with an uncomplicated pattern of gene regulation; (3) the fact that experience with HSCT demonstrates that the most severe manifestations of the disease can be corrected using ADA-replete hematopoietic cells; and (4) the poor outcomes in mismatched donor transplants. The advantages of GT over transplantation, which were stated then and which still hold true today, are that modification of autologous cells avoids the complications of graft-versus-host disease and because of the perceived survival advantage to ADA-replete cells, GT can be undertaken with little or no conditioning.

Several studies were conducted in the early 1990s, all of which used different forms of conventional gammaretroviral vectors encoding the ADA gene under the transcriptional control of the viral LTR (long terminal repeat).[38–41] The cellular target for the different studies varied from autologous peripheral blood lymphocytes (PBLs), to a combination of bone marrow and PBLs, to selected CD34+ stem cells from bone marrow or umbilical cord blood. In all these studies, no conditioning was given and all patients received PEG-ADA while undergoing GT. The major findings from these studies were that gene transfer into progenitor cell populations over extended time periods could be achieved and that there was little or no toxicity to patients as a result of gene transfer. However, no demonstrable improvement in immune function was seen as a result of the GT procedure.

It was not until early 2000s that more effective protocols were designed that eventually resulted in successful correction of the clinical and immunologic phenotype.[42–44] The major changes to the protocols were the withdrawal of PEG-ADA prior to the return of gene-transduced cells, thereby restoring a potential survival advantage to ADA-replete cells, and the use of mild nonmyeloablative conditioning to allow the long-term engraftment of a greater number of gene-modified cells at the outset. Trials in Milan and London, and a joint study between the Children's Hospital Los Angeles (CHLA) and the National Institutes of Health (NIH) treated a total of more than 20 patients. Each group used a different gammaretroviral vector and all transduced autologous selected CD34+ stem cells. The Milan and the United States studies used intravenous busulfan conditioning at a dose of approximately 4 mg/kg although the dosing regimes have varied between the 2 studies, and the London group used melphalan, 140 mg/kg, based on their experience of this chemotherapy regimen in their allogeneic transplant program.

The combined results from these 3 studies are very encouraging, and are summarized in **Table 1**. The majority of patients treated in these studies had previously shown an inadequate response to ERT or had failed an allogeneic transplant. In all patients, PEG-ADA was not given after the return of gene-modified cells. Following GT the majority of patients (67%) showed improved recovery of T-cell numbers compared with pre-GT levels. In these patients, it has not been necessary to restart ERT and several patients have remained off ERT for longer than 5 years, with the longest follow-up being approximately 8 years. Most impressively, all patients to date have survived the procedure and there have been no significant adverse events.

More detailed analysis of the data from these studies shows that T-cell recovery, although sufficient to protect individuals from infection, is at the lower end of the normal range. However, analysis of thymic function by TREC analysis or by surface phenotyping suggests that thymopoiesis is established in treated individuals and that T cells undergo thymic education before entering the peripheral circulation, suggesting that prethymic progenitors have been successfully transduced. These data are in keeping with the demonstration of a polyclonal T-cell repertoire and normal response to mitogenic and antigenic stimulation. Humoral function is less well reconstituted, although 5 of 10 children in the Milan study were able to discontinue immunoglobulin replacement therapy and showed vaccine-specific antibody responses.[44] The ability of patients to remain off ERT also demonstrates effective metabolic detoxification, and there is an impressive decrease in dATP levels. In some patients an increase in erythrocyte ADA levels was seen, indicating successful transduction of erythroid progenitors that were now capable of giving rise to ADA-replete red cells. Analysis of transgene levels showed that the majority of T and NK cells were gene marked, but also that there were lower but significant levels of marking in B cells and in the myeloid lineage.

GT in ADA-SCID has been highly successful, but these studies have run in parallel to studies of GT for SCID-X1[45,46] and X-linked chronic granulomatous disease (CGD).[47] In both latter studies, the success of GT has also been associated with gammaretroviral-mediated leukemogenesis.[47–49] Insertion of the gammaretroviral vector into the target cell chromosome is not a random process (as was thought at the initiation of these studies), and such vectors have a propensity to insert in and around the transcription start site of active genes. In 5 of 20 patients in studies of SCID-X1 and in 2 of 4 patients treated with GT for X-CGD, insertion of the vector into protooncogenes led to aberrant gene transcription of these genes and the proliferation of specific clones that eventually underwent leukemic transformation. Detailed analysis suggests that the powerful enhancer elements of the viral LTR were able to interact with nearby promoters, thereby activating aberrant protooncogene transcription. These

**Table 1**
**Summary of clinical trials of GT for ADA deficiency**

| Center | No. of Patients | Follow-Up (Years) | Off Enzyme | Survival | DFS |
|---|---|---|---|---|---|
| Milan | 10 | 1.8–8.0 | 8/10 | 100% | 80% |
| London | 6 | 1.0–6.0 | 3/6 | 100% | 50% |
| CHLA-NIH | 6 | 0.5–3 | 3/6 | 100% | 50% |
| UCLA-NIH | 3 | 0.1–0.5 | 3/3 | 100% | n.e. |
| Total | 25 | 0.1–8.0 | 17/25 | 100% | 67% |

*Abbreviations*: DFS, alive without bone marrow transplantation or PEG-ADA restart; n.e., not evaluable; UCLA, Unicersity of California, Los Angeles.

observations have naturally led to the analysis of retroviral integration sites in patients undergoing GT for ADA-SCID, and in keeping with findings from the other studies, vector integrations into or around protooncogenes have also been identified in ADA patients.[50,51] However, despite these similar integration profiles and similar duration of follow-up, no evidence of clonal dominance or proliferation has been observed in ADA-SCID patients. The reasons for these differing outcomes are difficult to explain, especially because the vector constructs and LTR sequences have in some cases been very similar and may indicate that GT for ADA-SCID has a more favorable risk profile, although extended follow-up is necessary before such statements can made more definitively. The observations do demand, however, that safety monitoring should be continued to be strictly implemented over the long term in all patients, according to guidelines of regulatory agencies. Further, the potential risks associated with the use of gammaretroviral vectors have led several groups to investigate the use self-inactivating vectors, such as lentiviral vectors,[52,53] which may in time improve the safety of GT for ADA-SCID.

## DISCUSSION

The data available from the 3 different therapeutic options have led to guidance on how to treat patients when faced with different donor availabilities. The initial stages for care of a child with ADA-SCID would be as for any child with SCID with treatment of active infection and stabilization of the clinical state, including optimal nutrition. In some cases and especially in infants with very poor nutrition or respiratory compromise, it may be advisable to start PEG-ADA to stabilize the child. Respiratory distress in an ADA-SCID child may in many cases be as a result of metabolic derangement rather than infection, and therefore detoxification with ERT may be acutely beneficial. As for other SCID forms, an urgent search for a donor should be undertaken.

If a fully matched sibling or family donor is available, the evidence currently available suggests that a transplant should be undertaken without any conditioning. The success rates associated with such procedures and the effective long-term reconstitution in both T- and B-cell compartments does not at present warrant the use of alternative therapies. Some have argued that the use of a conditioning regime may improve stem cell engraftment and promote an improved quality of immune reconstitution long term. However, the current data do not show any waning of immune function even more than 10 years after unconditioned HSCT, and the majority of patients have remained free of immunoglobulin therapy. Further strong evidence to the contrary would be required before this recommendation is changed. If PEG-ADA has been started, it is unlikely that there will have been significant immune recovery (which usually takes 3–6 months) before a matched sibling donor (MSD)/matched family donor (MFD) is found, in which case PEG-ADA can be stopped at the time of the unconditioned procedure.

If a matched MSD/MFD is unavailable, a search for an unrelated donor should be undertaken, during which time PEG-ADA should be started to promote improved nutrition and clinical well-being. If no matched donor is available, the transplant choice may be for a mismatched unrelated donor or a parental haploidentical donor transplant. The clear message from the currently available data is that these transplants are poorly tolerated and have a high degree of mortality in the conditioned setting as well as a high rate of rejection if performed without conditioning. For these reasons, it is advisable that these procedures are only undertaken if there is no access to ERT, perhaps for economic reasons, or if there is no possibility of enrolling the child into a trial of GT. Cord blood donations may tolerate a higher degree of HLA disparity, but there is currently insufficient evidence to inform any strong recommendation.

Therapeutic decision making is most problematic when faced with the choices of continuing ERT, undertaking a fully matched unrelated donor transplant, or enrolling the patient into a trial of GT. The continued administration of PEG-ADA represents the easiest and, in the short term, the safest choice. It is clear that patients benefit with clinical well-being, freedom from infection, and improved nutrition. However, the long-term data are fairly conclusive in showing that, over time, immune recovery is suboptimal and many children run very low T-cell numbers. Emerging reports documenting opportunistic infection in such individuals suggest that this option may not be beneficial long term, although it is difficult to specify the exact time period. The other concern is that the observed decrease in thymic function may ultimately limit the efficacy of a definitive procedure such as GT or allogeneic transplant. If physicians or parents are not keen to enter a definitive procedure initially and wish to continue ERT, a prudent approach may be to monitor patients carefully and at the first signs of waning T-cell or thymic function, consider the options of HSCT or GT. A further reason to discontinue ERT and offer HCT or GT would be the development of autoimmune cytopenias or neutralizing antibody that is refractory to immune modulation.

The choice between HSCT or GT as a definitive procedure is again difficult. Simply put, the choice may between the short-term risks associated with MUD HSCT against the potential for long-term side effects associated with GT. MUD HSCT has a 67% survival outcome given the present data, but this involves only 11 individuals. These figures may change significantly even if only a handful of further transplants are undertaken. It is clear, however, that outcome following these procedures is very good, with almost complete T- and B-cell reconstitution, and presently no evidence of long-term side effects. By contrast, GT has an excellent survival outcome and to date more than 20 children in 3 trials have survived the procedure without any significant side effects. The drawbacks of GT are twofold. First, there is the potential for insertional mutagenesis using the current vector technologies, although importantly the follow-up does not show any evidence of clonal proliferation in treated individuals. The other issue is that of immune recovery; at present 67% have been able to discontinue ERT on a long-term basis and approximately 50% have been able to discontinue Ig replacement. Thus the choice will eventually be determined by several factors, including the availability of the 2 modalities at treatment centers and, probably most importantly, the parental and physician attitude toward the risks and benefits associated with the 2 different treatment options.

This field is a rapidly evolving one. Advances in both HSCT- and GT-related technologies are likely to be implemented in the next few years and may greatly improve the safety profiles of these treatments. In HSCT, the use of newer chemotherapy agents such as treosulfan and the use of novel antibody-based conditioning agents[54] may reduce the toxicities associated with HSCT. Self-inactivating lentiviral vectors have already shown an improved safety profile in in vitro and in vivo models of stem cell transformation,[55,56] and if such safety improvements are demonstrated in clinical studies, this would represent a significant advance. Lentiviral vectors also show improved transduction of hematopoietic stem cells and preservation of stem cell capacity, which in turn may allow for improved ADA gene expression and immune recovery. Thus, the balance between these 2 modalities will need to be reviewed on a regular basis as results from the anticipated improvements emerge.

Further issues surround the best treatment for the nonimmunologic manifestations of ADA-SCID, and most importantly the cognitive and neurologic defects. At present, data are available only from those patients who have undergone HSCT, which highlights the incidence of mild to severe problems in this cohort. No data are available from patients undergoing ERT or GT. It may be hypothesized that better systemic detoxification may result in an amelioration of nonimmunologic abnormalities, and it will be important to formally study these patients. Such analysis is being planned. At present, however, these considerations cannot guide any specific treatment choice.

ADA-SCID is one of the most severe forms of SCID as a result of both the immunologic and metabolic abnormalities, and is a challenging disorder to treat. The availability of 3 different therapeutic options makes management decisions more difficult, but ultimately this does present choices that are not available for other SCID patients. Some strong recommendations can already be made based on current data and, as further developments in transplant and GT occur, it is likely that safer and more effective therapies will become available.

## ACKNOWLEDGMENTS

The author is supported in part by the Great Ormond Street Hospital Biomedical Research Center.

## REFERENCES

1. Hershfield MS, Mitchell BS. Immunodeficiency diseases caused by adenosine deaminase deficiency and purine nucleoside phosphorylase deficiency. In: Scriver CR, Beaudet AL, Sly WS, et al, editors. The metabolic and molecular basis of inherited disease. 7th edition. New York: McGraw-Hill; 1995. p. 1725–68.
2. Lee N, Russell N, Ganeshaguru K, et al. Mechanisms of deoxyadenosine toxicity in human lymphoid cells in vitro: relevance to the therapeutic use of inhibitors of adenosine deaminase. Br J Haematol 1984;56(1):107–19.
3. Apasov SG, Blackburn MR, Kellems RE, et al. Adenosine deaminase deficiency increases thymic apoptosis and causes defective T cell receptor signaling. J Clin Invest 2001;108(1):131–41.
4. Gangi-Peterson L, Sorscher DH, Reynolds JW, et al. Nucleotide pool imbalance and adenosine deaminase deficiency induce alterations of N-region insertions during V(D)J recombination. J Clin Invest 1999;103(6):833–41.
5. Benveniste P, Zhu W, Cohen A. Interference with thymocyte differentiation by an inhibitor of S-adenosylhomocysteine hydrolase. J Immunol 1995;155(2): 536–44.
6. Hershfield MS. New insights into adenosine-receptor-mediated immunosuppression and the role of adenosine in causing the immunodeficiency associated with adenosine deaminase deficiency. Eur J Immunol 2005;35(1):25–30.
7. Cassani B, Mirolo M, Cattaneo F, et al. Altered intracellular and extracellular signaling leads to impaired T-cell functions in ADA-SCID patients. Blood 2008; 111(8):4209–19.
8. Blackburn MR, Kellems RE. Adenosine deaminase deficiency: metabolic basis of immune deficiency and pulmonary inflammation. Adv Immunol 2005;86: 1–41.
9. Adams A, Harkness RA. Adenosine deaminase activity in thymus and other human tissues. Clin Exp Immunol 1976;26(3):647–9.
10. Van der Weyden MB, Kelley WN. Human adenosine deaminase. Distribution and properties. J Biol Chem 1976;251(18):5448–56.
11. Carson DA, Kaye J, Seegmiller JE. Lymphospecific toxicity in adenosine deaminase deficiency and purine nucleoside phosphorylase deficiency: possible role of nucleoside kinase(s). Proc Natl Acad Sci U S A 1977;74(12):5677–81.

12. Cederbaum SD, Kaitila I, Rimoin DL, et al. The chondro-osseous dysplasia of adenosine deaminase deficiency with severe combined immunodeficiency. J Pediatr 1976;89(5):737–42.

13. Hirschhorn R, Paageorgiou PS, Kesarwala HH, et al. Amelioration of neurologic abnormalities after "enzyme replacement" in adenosine deaminase deficiency. N Engl J Med 1980;303(7):377–80.

14. Rogers MH, Lwin R, Fairbanks L, et al. Cognitive and behavioral abnormalities in adenosine deaminase deficient severe combined immunodeficiency. J Pediatr 2001;139(1):44–50.

15. Titman P, Pink E, Skucek E, et al. Cognitive and behavioral abnormalities in children after hematopoietic stem cell transplantation for severe congenital immunodeficiencies. Blood 2008;112(9):3907–13.

16. Albuquerque W, Gaspar HB. Bilateral sensorineural deafness in adenosine deaminase-deficient severe combined immunodeficiency. J Pediatr 2004;144(2):278–80.

17. Bollinger ME, Arredondo-Vega FX, Santisteban I, et al. Brief report: hepatic dysfunction as a complication of adenosine deaminase deficiency. N Engl J Med 1996;334(21):1367–71.

18. Migchielson AAJ, Breuer ML, van Roon MA, et al. Adenosine-deaminase-deficient mice die perinatally and exhibit liver-cell degeneration, atelectasis and small intestinal cell death. Nat Genet 1996;10:279–87.

19. Wakamiya M, Blackburn MR, Jurecic R, et al. Disruption of the adenosine deaminase gene causes hepatocellular impairment and perinatal lethality in mice. Proc Natl Acad Sci U S A 1995;92(9):3673–7.

20. Blackburn MR, Datta SK, Kellems RE. Adenosine deaminase-deficient mice generated using a two-stage genetic engineering strategy exhibit a combined immunodeficiency. J Biol Chem 1998;273(9):5093–100.

21. Turner CP, Seli M, Ment L, et al. A1 adenosine receptors mediate hypoxia-induced ventriculomegaly. Proc Natl Acad Sci U S A 2003;100(20):11718–22.

22. Antoine C, Muller S, Cant A, et al. Long-term survival and transplantation of haemopoietic stem cells for immunodeficiencies: report of the European experience 1968-99. Lancet 2003;361(9357):553–60.

23. Grunebaum E, Mazzolari E, Porta F, et al. Bone marrow transplantation for severe combined immune deficiency. JAMA 2006;295(5):508–18.

24. Gaspar HB, Aiuti A, Porta F, et al. How I treat ADA deficiency. Blood 2009;114(17):3524–32.

25. Booth C, Hershfield M, Notarangelo L, et al. Management options for adenosine deaminase deficiency; proceedings of the EBMT satellite workshop (Hamburg, March 2006). Clin Immunol 2007;123(2):139–47.

26. Carbonaro DA, Jin X, Cotoi D, et al. Neonatal bone marrow transplantation of ADA-deficient SCID mice results in immunologic reconstitution despite low levels of engraftment and an absence of selective donor T lymphoid expansion. Blood 2008;111(12):5745–54.

27. Abuchowski A, McCoy JR, Palczuk NC, et al. Effect of covalent attachment of polyethylene glycol on immunogenicity and circulating life of bovine liver catalase. J Biol Chem 1977;252(11):3582–6.

28. Davis S, Abuchowski A, Park YK, et al. Alteration of the circulating life and antigenic properties of bovine adenosine deaminase in mice by attachment of polyethylene glycol. Clin Exp Immunol 1981;46:649–52.

29. Hershfield MS, Chaffee S, Sorensen RU. Enzyme replacement therapy with polyethylene glycol-adenosine deaminase in adenosine deaminase deficiency: overview

and case reports of three patients, including two now receiving gene therapy. Pediatr Res 1993;33(1 Suppl):S42–7.

30. Hershfield MS. PEG-ADA replacement therapy for adenosine deaminase deficiency: an update after 8.5 years. Clin Immunol Immunopathol 1995;76(3 Pt 2): S228–32.

31. Hershfield MS. Combined immune deficiencies due to purine enzyme defects. In: Steim ER, Ochs HD, Winkelstein JA, editors. Immunologic disorders in infants and children. Philadelphia: W.B.Saunders; 2004. p. 480–504.

32. Malacarne F, Benicchi T, Notarangelo LD, et al. Reduced thymic output, increased spontaneous apoptosis and oligoclonal B cells in polyethylene glycol-adenosine deaminase-treated patients. Eur J Immunol 2005;35(11): 3376–86.

33. Chan B, Wara D, Bastian J, et al. Long-term efficacy of enzyme replacement therapy for adenosine deaminase (ADA)-deficient severe combined immunodeficiency (SCID). Clin Immunol 2005;117(2):133–43.

34. Husain M, Grunebaum E, Naqvi A, et al. Burkitt's lymphoma in a patient with adenosine deaminase deficiency-severe combined immunodeficiency treated with polyethylene glycol-adenosine deaminase. J Pediatr 2007;151(1):93–5.

35. Kaufman DA, Hershfield MS, Bocchini JA, et al. Cerebral lymphoma in an adenosine deaminase-deficient patient with severe combined immunodeficiency receiving polyethylene glycol-conjugated adenosine deaminase. Pediatrics 2005;116(6):e876–9.

36. Lainka E, Hershfield MS, Santisteban I, et al. polyethylene glycol-conjugated adenosine deaminase (ADA) therapy provides temporary immune reconstitution to a child with delayed-onset ADA deficiency. Clin Diagn Lab Immunol 2005; 12(7):861–6.

37. Chaffee S, Mary A, Stiehm ER, et al. IgG antibody response to polyethylene glycol-modified adenosine deaminase in patients with adenosine deaminase deficiency. J Clin Invest 1992;89(5):1643–51.

38. Blaese RM, Culver KW, Miller AD, et al. T lymphocyte-directed gene therapy for ADA-SCID: initial trial results after 4 years. Science 1995;270:475–80.

39. Bordignon C, Notarangelo LD, Nobili N, et al. Gene therapy in peripheral blood lymphocytes and bone marrow for ADA- immunodeficient patients. Science 1995;270(5235):470–5.

40. Kohn DB, Weinberg KI, Nolta JA, et al. Engraftment of gene-modified umbilical cord blood cells in neonates with adenosine deaminase deficiency. Nat Med 1995;1(10):1017–23.

41. Hoogerbrugge PM, van Beusechem VW, Fischer A, et al. Bone marrow gene transfer in three patients with adenosine deaminase deficiency. Gene Ther 1996;3:179–83.

42. Aiuti A, Slavin S, Aker M, et al. Correction of ADA-SCID by stem cell gene therapy combined with nonmyeloablative conditioning. Science 2002;296(5577): 2410–3.

43. Gaspar HB, Bjorkegren E, Parsley K, et al. Successful reconstitution of immunity in ADA-SCID by stem cell gene therapy following cessation of PEG-ADA and use of mild preconditioning. Mol Ther 2006;14(4):505–13.

44. Aiuti A, Cattaneo F, Galimberti S, et al. Gene therapy for immunodeficiency due to adenosine deaminase deficiency. N Engl J Med 2009;360(5):447–58.

45. Cavazzana-Calvo M, Hacein-Bey S, de Saint BG, et al. Gene therapy of human severe combined immunodeficiency (SCID)-X1 disease. Science 2000;288(5466): 669–72.

46. Gaspar HB, Parsley KL, Howe S, et al. Gene therapy of X-linked severe combined immunodeficiency by use of a pseudotyped gammaretroviral vector. Lancet 2004;364(9452):2181–7.

47. Ott MG, Schmidt M, Schwarzwaelder K, et al. Correction of X-linked chronic granulomatous disease by gene therapy, augmented by insertional activation of MDS1-EVI1, PRDM16 or SETBP1. Nat Med 2006;12(4):401–9.

48. Hacein-Bey-Abina S, von Kalle C, Schmidt M, et al. LMO2-associated clonal T cell proliferation in two patients after gene therapy for SCID-X1. Science 2003; 302(5644):415–9.

49. Howe SJ, Mansour MR, Schwarzwaelder K, et al. Insertional mutagenesis combined with acquired somatic mutations causes leukemogenesis following gene therapy of SCID-X1 patients. J Clin Invest 2008;118(9):3143–50.

50. Aiuti A, Cassani B, Andolfi G, et al. Multilineage hematopoietic reconstitution without clonal selection in ADA-SCID patients treated with stem cell gene therapy. J Clin Invest 2007;117(8):2233–40.

51. Cassani B, Montini E, Maruggi G, et al. Integration of retroviral vectors induces minor changes in the transcriptional activity of T cells from ADA-SCID patients treated with gene therapy. Blood 2009;114(17):3546–56.

52. Mortellaro A, Hernandez RJ, Guerrini MM, et al. Ex vivo gene therapy with lentiviral vectors rescues adenosine deaminase (ADA)-deficient mice and corrects their immune and metabolic defects. Blood 2006;108(9):2979–88.

53. Carbonaro DA, Jin X, Petersen D, et al. In vivo transduction by intravenous injection of a lentiviral vector expressing human ADA into neonatal ADA gene knockout mice: a novel form of enzyme replacement therapy for ADA deficiency. Mol Ther 2006;13(6):1110–20.

54. Straathof KC, Rao K, Eyrich M, et al. Haemopoietic stem-cell transplantation with antibody-based minimal-intensity conditioning: a phase 1/2 study. Lancet 2009; 374(9693):912–20.

55. Modlich U, Navarro S, Zychlinski D, et al. Insertional transformation of hematopoietic cells by self-inactivating lentiviral and gammaretroviral vectors. Mol Ther 2009;17(11):1919–28.

56. Montini E, Cesana D, Schmidt M, et al. Hematopoietic stem cell gene transfer in a tumor-prone mouse model uncovers low genotoxicity of lentiviral vector integration. Nat Biotechnol 2006;24(6):687–96.

# Gene Therapy for Primary Immunodeficiencies

Alain Fischer, MD, PhD[a,b,c,]*, S. Hacein-Bey-Abina, PharmD, PhD[a,b,d,e],
M. Cavazanna-Calvo, MD, PhD[a,b,d,e]

**KEYWORDS**

- Severe combined immunodeficiencies • Gene therapy
- Hematopoietic stem cells • Retrovirus • Lentivirus
- Wiskott Aldrich • Chronic granulomatous disease • Clinical trial

The concept of gene therapy emerged as a way of correcting monogenic inherited diseases by introducing a normal copy of the mutated gene into at least some of the patients' cells.[1] Although this concept has turned out to be quite complicated to implement, it is in the field of primary immunodeficiencies (PIDs) that proof of feasibility has been undoubtedly achieved. There is now a strong rationale in support of gene therapy for at least some PIDs, as discussed later in this article.

## RATIONALE

Many PIDs are lethal diseases. In the absence of treatment, severe combined immunodeficiencies (SCIDs) cause death within the first year of life. Many other combined deficiencies of adaptive immunity (such as Wiskott Aldrich syndrome [WAS] and diseases causing hemophagocytic lymphohistiocytosis [HLH]) can also be fatal in young infants. Allogeneic hematopoietic stem cell transplantation (HSCT) can cure many of these disorders by replacing the diseased hematopoietic lineages with normal ones.[2] These results prove that transplantation of normal hematopoietic stem cells or their progenitors can correct a large variety of PIDs of the adaptive and innate immune systems. However, HSCT is associated with several serious adverse events, including

[a] Developpement Normal et Pathologique du Systeme Immunitaire, INSERM U 768, Hopital Necker, 149 rue de sevres, Paris 75015, France
[b] Paris-Descartes University, Hopital Necker, 149 rue de sevres, Paris 75015, France
[c] Unité d'Immunologie et Hématologie Pédiatrique, Assistance Publique, Hôpital Necker Enfants Malades, Hopital Necker, 149 rue de sevres, Paris 75015, France
[d] Department of Biotherapy, Hopital Necker-Enfants Malades, Assistance Publique-Hôpitaux de Paris (AP-HP), Université René Descartes, Hopital Necker, 149 rue de sevres, Paris 75015, France
[e] INSERM, Centre d'Investigation Clinique intégré en Biothérapies, Groupe Hospitalier Universitaire Ouest, AP-HP, Hopital Necker, 149 rue de sevres, Paris 75015, France
* Corresponding author. Developpement Normal et Pathologique du Systeme Immunitaire, INSERM U 768, Hopital Necker, 149 rue de sevres, Paris 75015, France.
*E-mail address:* alain.fischer@inserm.fr

the toxicity of myeloablative chemotherapy and, above all, the consequences of the potential immune conflict between donor and recipient. The latter can result in either graft failure or, conversely, graft-versus-host disease, a cause of serious morbidity and mortality.[3] In the context of human leukocyte antigen (HLA) mismatch, the risk for immune conflict can be alleviated by removing donor T cells from the stem cell inoculum. However, this type of approach is still marred by the risk for graft failure and prolonged immunodeficiency before donor-derived immunity develops. Although advances in HSCT methodology may provide better solutions to these problems,[4] it is clearly legitimate to search for alternative, gene-based approaches.

Most PIDs display Mendelian inheritance, so that addition of a normal copy of the mutated gene can correct the deficiency provided that the right cells are targeted and transgene expression is appropriate. At present, the pathophysiological mechanisms of many PIDs have been worked out and provide further clues to the use of gene therapy.

Information on gene expression pattern and regulation is essential for assessing the therapeutic feasibility. For instance, the tightly regulated expression of CD40L (the protein that is deficient in X-linked hyper IgM syndrome) precludes gene therapy in its present form because such precise regulatory control cannot yet be mimicked. Indeed, continuous expression of CD40L led to the development of lymphoma when tested in CD40L-deficient mice.[5] Given that several of the genes mutated in PIDs encode proteins involved in cell survival/proliferation, their expression is expected to provide a significant growth advantage over non-corrected cells during differentiation (see later discussion). This key point was eventually verified in the first successful clinical trials.

While the pathophysiology of many PIDs was being deciphered, significant advances were also made in the development of vectors capable of efficiently transducing mature lymphocytes and progenitor cells. These new vectors (γ retroviruses, lentiviruses, spumaviruses, and possibly retrotransposons) are all characterized by their ability to integrate into the host genome so that the therapeutic transgene is replicated during cell division and thus is stably transmitted to the progeny.[6] This property is mandatory for gene therapy in mitotic cells, such as immune cell precursors and mature lymphocytes. Initial attempts used the long terminal repeat (LTR) of retroviruses as a promoter, whereas progress toward the use of internal promoters in conjunction with deletion of the LTR enhancer activity (the so-called self-inactivated LTR [SIN-LTR]) were made to promote safety (see later discussion).[7] Furthermore, the technical aspects of ex vivo gene transfer into hematopoietic progenitors have been improved over the years by using appropriate cytokine cocktails to put cells in cycle retrovirus (RV) or in G1 of the cell cycle lentivirus (LV) and thus facilitate vector integration. Use of fibronectin fragments also promotes cell infection by vectors. These developments made gene therapy a feasible option for some PIDs at least.[6]

## GENE THERAPY FOR SEVERE COMBINED IMMUNODEFICIENCIES -X1

The most frequent SCID is SCID-X1; the condition is caused by a deficiency in the common γc cytokine receptor subunit, which causes a complete block in T-cell and Natural killer (NK)-cell development.[8] It was first thought that SCID-X1 was the most accurate model for assessing gene therapy because spontaneous reversion of the mutation in the γc-encoding IL2RG gene led to significant correction of the immune deficiency. This observation supported the hypothesis whereby transduced lymphocyte progenitors have a selective advantage over their non-transduced counterparts.[9] Furthermore, IL2RG is expressed by all hematopoietic cells and is not tightly regulated, thus reducing the risk for toxicity related to aberrant expression. It was thus expected that gene correction of a proportion of lymphoid progenitors would be enough to restore at least the T-cell compartment and that the effect would be long lasting (because T cells live for several decades).

Thus, following in vitro and in vivo preclinical tests in $\gamma$c-deficient mice, clinical trials were designed. The vectors were based on the use of RV constructs in which IL2GR was placed under the transcriptional control of the LTR, with the use of either an amphotropic envelope[10] or the gibbon ape leukemia virus envelope.[11] Between 1999 and 2006, 20 subjects with archetypal SCID-X1 were treated in two trials in Paris and then London.[10–15] All the subjects lacked an HLA-identical donor. They received ex vivo transduced CD34 cells in the absence of any additional therapy. The outcome of these trials (in toxicity and then efficacy) can be summarized as follows. Five of the 20 subjects developed T-cell leukemia 2.5 to 5 years after gene therapy.[14,16,17] In four cases, chemotherapy was easily able to destroy abnormal clones so that these children are currently in remission and doing well. However, despite chemotherapy, the one remaining subject died from refractory leukemia.[17] The occurrence of these complications was serious enough to prompt discontinuation of the trials. Considerable efforts were made to understand the mechanism by which (with an unexpectedly high frequency) this complication had occurred. It was found that proliferative clones carried RV integrations within oncogenes loci.[14,17] One oncogene in particular (LMO-2) was targeted in four out five cases. Integration of the vector containing a functional LTR enhancer had led to uncontrolled expression activity of the oncogenes.[14,16,17] Secondary genomic modifications, such as loss of the p19Arf locus and NOTCH1-activating mutations, contributed to the clonal selection. It was then realized that the pattern of RV integration was, in contrast to previous hypotheses, semi-random with selective integration into gene loci (60% of all integrations) equally distributed between regulatory sequences 5' from the transcription start site and the gene itself (including the first few introns).[18] Furthermore, integrations were more frequent in genes being actively expressed in the target cells, as it is the case for several proto-oncogenes (including LMO-2) in hematopoietic progenitor cells.[14,16,17] It thus became clear that RV-mediated gene transfer could deregulate proto-oncogene expression through the LTRs enhancer activity. It is nevertheless likely that additional factors are involved, because none of the 14 subjects successfully treated with a similar gene-therapy approach for another SCID (adenosine deaminase [ADA] deficiency,[19] see later discussion) developed leukemic complications, despite the fact that a similar RV integrations pattern was found.[20,21] These observations suggest that either $\gamma$c expression by lymphoid progenitors exerts some form of synergistic effect with oncogene deregulation (although there is no evidence of $\gamma$c overexpression or active downstream signaling) or that an impairment in progenitor cell distribution caused by $\gamma$c or ADA deficiency influences the risk for oncogene transactivation.

Indeed, progenitor cells differ in their sensitivity to transformation, perhaps because of gene expression or activation or the cell cycle patterns. These considerations are obviously of the utmost importance for further assessment of the risk associated with gene therapy. At present, there is a consensus that use of SIN vectors featuring an internal promoter with weak enhancer activity should reduce this risk. Although this is supported by in vitro experiments,[22] the available in vivo experimental models do not yet constitute a sufficiently predictive toxicity assay despite considerable experimental efforts.[23,24] Further safety measures include the presence of insulators in the vector (to prevent the transactivation of neighboring genes) and the potential addition of a suicide gene.[25,26] However, none of these modifications are likely to be absolute solutions and may carry disadvantages.

Lentiviral vectors based on HIV might be safer because they do not target 5' regu-latory responses.[27] However, they still integrate into genes. Given the overall higher transduction efficiency of LV (as based on the number of integration sites in progenitor cells), LV and RV vectors do not greatly differ in oncogenicity.[28] Spumaviruses may also be of value because they integrate into genes less frequently than RVs and LVs do.[29] Nevertheless, significant issues in vector production must be solved before the effective use of spumaviruses can be envisaged.

The efficacy of γc gene transfer has been clearly demonstrated. Between 4 and 10.5 years after gene therapy, 17 of the 20 subjects are alive and display full or nearly full correction of the T-cell immunodeficiency[10,12,14]: T-cell subset counts, sustained detection of naive T cells (even in the subjects who had been treated for leukemia), a diversified T-cell repertoire, and T-cell–mediated immune functions. The γc gene transfer led to clear clinical benefits, because patients first recovered from ongoing infections with a poor prognosis and were then able to live in a normal environment without any evidence of particular susceptibilities to infection. The extent of correction of the NK-cell deficiency was not as impressive. Despite an early rise, NK-cell counts eventually dropped to low values. Remarkably, this was also observed in patients with non-myeloablated SCID-X1 who had undergone allogeneic HSCT. A partially persis-tent NK-cell deficiency does not appear to be harmful. This finding indicates that NK-cell population dynamics (cell development, expansion, and survival) differ signif-icantly from those of T cells. The frequency of transduced B cells was low (<1%) and these cells were no longer detected in the blood 2 to 3 years after gene therapy. This observation emphasizes the lack of persistence of transduced progenitors in the bone marrow. In contrast, the sustained detection of naive T cells (even in patients having undergone chemotherapy for leukemia) strongly suggests the persistence of trans-duced (T) cell precursors that have perhaps localized in the thymus. Despite the apparent lack of persistent γc[+] B cells, most patients do not require immunoglobulin substitution. Overall, these results constitute the first proof of principle of gene therapy and its sustained efficacy. As anticipated in this context, efficacy is based on the selective advantage provided by γc expression in lymphoid progenitors. These data pave the way for further use of gene therapy in patients with SCID-X1, as now sched-uled in an international trial (in the United Kingdom, United States, and France) using SIN vectors. Similar attempts have been made to treat patients with atypical SCID-X1 (caused by hypomorphic mutations) or those who displayed limited T-cell reconstitu-tion following HSCT. Effective CD34-cell transduction resulted in little or no improve-ment in T-cell production, probably as a consequence of thymic function loss.[30,31] This parameter must therefore also be taken into account when considering gene therapy in patients who are T-cell deficient after the first few years of life.

## GENE THERAPY FOR ADENOSINE DEAMINASE DEFICIENCY

Adenosine deaminase deficiency is a rare, autosomal recessive PID characterized by a profound impairment in the generation of T, B, and NK lymphocytes. It is thus a partic-ularly severe form of SCID, with early onset of infectious complications.[32] Adenosine deaminase deficiency results in a purine metabolism defect; the accumulation of aden-osine, deoxyadenosine and their metabolites (notably deoxyadenosine triphosphate [dATP]) induces the premature death of lymphoid progenitor cells. It is a disease with broad consequences, because ADA deficiency also impairs (to a varying extent) bone, brain, lungs, liver functions and perhaps the epithelia. It is thus one of the SCIDs with the worst overall prognosis. Adenosine deaminase deficiency was the first PID in which gene therapy was tested. The initial approach was ex vivo ADA gene transfer into peripheral T cells that were obtained from patients undergoing enzyme substitution therapy. Although this approach failed to reconstitute immunity, it demonstrated the feasibility of gene transfer and the long-term viability (>10 years) of transduced CD8 T cells at least in one subject.[33] Adenosine deaminase deficiency was also the first PID in which researchers tested ex vivo ADA gene transfer mediated by an RV vector in CD34 progenitor cells from bone marrow and cord blood.[34,35] At that time, gene-transfer technology was not efficient enough to ensure sufficient progenitor cell transduction and correction of the PID. Nevertheless, long-term detection of a few transduced T cells was confirmed.[36,37] Concomitant enzyme substitution therapy also optimally reduced the transduced cells' selective advantage.

In the modern era of gene therapy, efficient ex vivo ADA gene transfer mediated by an RV vector in CD34 cells has been achieved. When combined with a partially myeloablative conditioning regimen (4 mg/kg busulfan), this protocol corrected the PID in 14 out of 20 patients treated once enzyme substitution had been withdrawn (or was not initiated).[19,38] Sustained correction has now been observed for up to 8 years, with clear-cut clinical benefits and no toxicity (see earlier discussion). Because of the administration of busulfan, it was found that transduced cells were detectable not only in T populations (all of which were transduced) but also in NK, B, and myeloid populations. The degree of T-cell correction in ADA deficiency does not appear to be as complete as in SCID-X1; this is probably a consequence of additional effects of ADA deficiency, such as damage to the thymic epithelium, that are not amenable to correction by ex vivo gene transfer into CD34 cells. In any case, the reproducible, sustained correction of the consequences of immunodeficiency in two SCIDs clearly proves the feasibility of this approach and suggests that, provided oncogene transactivation can be prevented, ex vivo gene transfer is an alternative to HSCT in the absence of available HLA-identical donors.

## GENE THERAPY FOR OTHER SEVERE COMBINED IMMUNODEFICIENCIES AND OTHER SEVERE T-CELL IMMUNODEFICIENCIES

Fifteen distinct genetic defects have been found in association with SCID.[39] These conditions are all potential candidates for gene therapy, although the extreme rarity of some of them may hamper efforts to develop an appropriate vector up to the clinical phase. At the preclinical level, gene transfer efficacy has been shown for Rag-2, Artemis, JAK3, and ZAP70 deficiencies.[40–44] A clinical trial for the T- B- SCID condition caused by Artemis deficiency is being planned. An interesting strategy has been tested in a murine model of ZAP70 deficiency, with direct, intrathymic injection of the RV vector.[44] This treatment led to significant correction of the immunodeficiency, although it is not known whether this approach will enable the sufficiently long-term persistence of transduced progenitors. Furthermore, in humans, the accessibility of the T-cell–devoid thymus is questionable. For unknown reasons, it has not yet been possible to achieve reproducible, sustained correction of Rag-1 deficiency in mice without using a high vector multiplicity of infection to achieve integration of multiple copies per transduced cell, which is a setting with a high risk for insertional mutagenesis and oncogene transactivation.[45]

## GENE THERAPY FOR WISKOTT ALDRICH SYNDROME

Wiskott Aldrich syndrome is an X-linked condition characterized by a multicell immunodeficiency that affects at least T and B lymphocytes and dendritic cells and by a thrombocytopenia. It is caused by loss-of-function mutations in the WAS protein (WASp) gene,[46] which is usually ubiquitously expressed within the hematopoietic system. When activated, WASp regulates the actin cytoskeleton. A WASp deficiency induces multiple defects in cell migration, activation, and survival. The severity of WAS depends on the type of mutation. Severe forms are life-threatening in childhood because of vulnerability to several pathogens associated with the onset of severe autoimmune manifestations, and in some cases, tumors. Following fully or partially myeloablative chemotherapy, allogeneic HSCT can cure WAS. The outcome for HSCT from HLA identical donors is good, whereas mortality is high in other settings. This is why several groups have considered WAS as a good candidate for gene therapy. RV and LV vectors are able to transduce WASp-deficient murine progenitor cells and correct (mild) WAS disease in mice.[47,48] Furthermore, in vitro experiments have shown that transduced human T cells and dendritic cells can be generated and recover normal functions.[49–51] Of particular interest is the LV vector in which the endogenous WASP promoter is being used to drive WASp expression at a physiologic level.[51] It is expected that transduced CD34 cells should have some degree of selective advantage over non-transduced cells, which facilitates clinical efficacy. The first clinical trial, based on a conventional RV vector with the WASP gene under the control of the LTR, has been initiated. After partially myeloablative conditioning, CD34 cells are ex vivo transduced and reinjected.[52] Although the preliminary data (after 2 to 3 years of follow-up) suggest that the manifestations of WAS have been effectively corrected, the safety concern is still to be addressed. Trials based on the use of a SIN LV vector with the endogenous WASP promoter are being planned. One possible concern for the long-term efficacy of gene therapy for WAS (and HSCT, in fact) stems from the observation that patients with WAS having undergone allogeneic HSCT are at a greater risk for relapse of autoimmune manifestations if autologous B cells persist post-HSCT.[53]

## GENE THERAPY FOR OTHER PRIMARY IMMUNODEFICIENCIES OF THE ADAPTIVE IMMUNE SYSTEM

Hemophagocytic lymphohistiocytosis (HLH) is a condition generated by a group of genetic diseases (notably perforin, Munc13-4, Rab27a, Syntaxin11, Munc18-2, and SH2DIA deficiencies) in which cytotoxic lymphocyte function is impaired.[54] The condition is fatal in the absence of therapy and can be cured by allogeneic HSCT. Two gene-therapy strategies can be considered here: ex vivo gene transfer into peripheral CD8 T cells (to restore cytotoxic function) or CD34+ progenitor cells. The first scenario has some advantages: RV (LV)-mediated transfer into T cells is safe[55] and does not require prior myeloablation of the patients (in contrast to the HSCT approach). However, it might be difficult to tailor the efficacy of therapy in transduced CD8 T cells to be injected and the frequency of repeat injections. Relevant murine models might address these questions to some extent.

Similarly, immunoproliferative, entheropathy X-linked (IPEX) syndrome is a very severe condition that results in defective FOXP3 CD4+ CD25+ regulatory T cells. It is caused by loss-of-function mutations in the gene encoding FOXP3.[56] The syndrome is characterized by devastating, early-onset inflammation of the gut, which is often associated with diabetes, autoimmune cytopenia, and severe skin allergies. Hematopoietic stem-cell transplantation can cure IPEX, although reports of success are still scarce. Ex vivo transduction of CD4 T cells (leading to FOXP3 expression) would be an elegant and probably nontoxic approach for generating regulatory T cells able to control disease manifestations. There are, however, several questions to be solved before clinical applications can be envisaged (as is also the case for HLH): the number of cells to be injected, the control of FOXP3 expression, the injection frequency, and the quality of the in vivo function in the induced regulatory T cells.

B-cell immunodeficiencies could also be candidates for gene therapy. X-L agam-maglobulinemia (XLA) has been considered as a model, because transduction of bone marrow progenitors with a vector carrying the BTK gene (which is mutated in XLA) could restore B-cell differentiation.[57] However, XLA is not as life threatening as the PIDs discussed earlier and so safety issues would have to be completely solved before clinical trials are initiated. In particular, BTK expression should be restricted to B cells (monocytes and mast cells) to avoid possible toxicity (over activation?) of cells in which BTK is not usually expressed, such as T lymphocytes.

## GENE THERAPY FOR CHRONIC GRANULOMATOUS DISEASE

Chronic granulomatous disease (CGD) is an inherited (X-linked or autosomal reces-sive) condition characterized by defective killing of bacteria and fungi by neutrophils and monocytes/macrophages because of defective generation of reactive oxygen species in the phagosome membrane.[58] Life-threatening infections and chronic inflammation are the main consequences of this defect. Mutations in five genes encoding various components of nicotinamide adenine dinucleotide phosphate (NADPH) oxidase have been described in patients with CGD.

The most frequent form of CGD is X-linked and is caused by a lack of the gp91 phox protein. At present, patients with poor infection control are treated (with some success) with allogeneic HSCT. Hence, there is a rationale for a gene-therapy approach, although, unlike what was observed in SCID and is generally expected in WAS, expression of gp91 phox or the other defective proteins in myeloid precursor cells is not going to provide a selective advantage. Furthermore, the short life span of neutrophils (around 2 days) implies that a large number of stem cells will have to be transduced to ensure the long-term production of corrected neutrophils and mono-cytes. Thus, CGD is a tough candidate for gene therapy. The approach will require a combination of fully myeloablative conditioning and efficient transduction of stem cells (probably with LV vectors). This hypothesis was confirmed by the outcome of the first clinical trial of CGD gene therapy performed in the absence of myeloablation. Only low (<1%) levels of transduced neutrophils were transiently detected.[59] More recently, Grez and colleagues reported the apparently efficient correction of CGD in two adult subjects who had received myeloablative conditioning. Gene transfer of the gp91 phox-encoding gene was mediated by using an RV vector with a strong ability to induce gene expression in myeloid cells (spleen focus-forming virus [SFFV] LTR).[60] In both subjects, progressive accumulation of transduced neutrophils and monocytes in the blood was observed over the first few months post-injection. Restored NADPH oxidase activity was found on these cells. Clinical benefit was observed, because the subjects managed to clear concurrent chest *Aspergillus* infec-tions. It was found that myelopoiesis was oligoclonal and driven by clones in which the vector had integrated near to three known oncogenes (Evi-1, PRD1M16, and STBP1). These oncogenes had been transactivated and thus provided the clones serendipi-tously with a selective advantage. Unfortunately, a myelodysplastic syndrome devel-oped and was associated (in one subject) with extinction of transgene expression and a fatal outcome.[61] This observation also highlights the importance of the selective advantage that can be conferred by either transgene expression (in SCID, for example) or transactivation of an endogenous gene (leukemia in SCID-X1 and CGD). Further developments of gene therapy for CGD[62] will thus have to combine full myeloablative chemotherapy (to get rid of several non-transduced cells) and ex vivo gene transfer into HSCs by using a SIN LV vector. It was recently reported that the same approach gave stable transgene expression (more than 3 years, to date) in hematopoietic lineages in three subjects with adrenoleukodystrophy.[63] The transgene is expressed by about 10% to 15% of blood cells, which is a proportion that would be sufficient to clear CGD symptoms. Thus, the experience gathered in this non-PID model is encouraging for use of gene therapy for PIDs of the innate immune system, such as CGD and perhaps also leukocyte adhesion deficiency. The latter disease was reportedly cured in a murine model by using ex vivo β2 integrin gene transfer with a spumavirus vector.[64]

## SUMMARY

The last decade has witnessed the effective advent of gene therapy as a treatment for two severe PIDs. Provided that safety issues can be mastered, today's technology opens the way to applying gene therapy to several life-threatening PIDs, including those in which transduction with the transgene does not provide a selective advantage. There will be several mandatory conditions: a carefully designed clinical research protocol, extensive monitoring of enrolled subjects, and real-time access to the results for the whole community to adjust practice worldwide and limit the occurrence of adverse events. Given the extensive requirements of these approaches, international collaborations are needed. Further progress can be expected. For example, PIDs caused by dominant mutations with negative effects, such as autoimmune lymphoproliferative syndrome or certain interferon γ, receptor deficiencies, could be treated by allele-specific oligonucleotide transfer, inducing degradation of the mutated allele.[65] Some mutations in complex genes with multiple exons might be treated by the exon-skipping methodology that is presently being tested in certain forms of Duchenne muscular dystrophy.[66]

Potentially, gene transfer could be targeted to a safe harbor in a genome area devoid of oncogenes.[67] An initial approach using bacterial integrases turned out to be cytotoxic but technology based on homologous recombination with engineered endonucleases (Zinc finger nucleases or meganucleases derived from the yeast Isce-1 endonuclease) might be useable.[68,69] The same approach could also be used for direct mutated gene repair by providing a template for homologous recombination.[69] This approach was effective for IL2RG in certain cell lines, although potential off-target action and the efficacy of homologous recombination in stem cells remain significant hurdles.

As was the case for HSCT, PIDs are at the forefront of development efforts in gene therapy. It is likely that during the next decade we shall see a significant shift toward gene therapy in the treatment of several PIDs.

## ACKNOWLEDGMENTS

The authors are grateful to Malika Tiouri-Sifouane for her excellent secretarial assistance.

## REFERENCES

1. Friedmann T, Roblin R. Gene therapy for human genetic disease? Science 1972; 175(25):949–55.
2. Antoine C, Muller S, Cant A, et al. Long-term survival and transplantation of haemopoietic stem cells for immunodeficiencies: report of the European experience 1968–99. Lancet 2003;361(9357):553–60.

3. Socie G, Blazar BR. Acute graft-versus-host disease: from the bench to the bedside. Blood 2009;114(20):4327–36.
4. Hagin D, Reisner Y. Haploidentical bone marrow transplantation in primary immune deficiency: stem cell selection and manipulation. Immunol Allergy Clin North Am 2010;30(1):45–62.
5. Brown MP, Topham DJ, Sangster MY, et al. Thymic lymphoproliferative disease after successful correction of CD40 ligand deficiency by gene transfer in mice. Nat Med 1998;4(11):1253–60.
6. Verma IM, Weitzman MD. Gene therapy: twenty-first century medicine. Annu Rev Biochem 2005;74:711–38.
7. Yu SF, von Ruden T, Kantoff PW, et al. Self-inactivating retroviral vectors designed for transfer of whole genes into mammalian cells. Proc Natl Acad Sci U S A 1986; 83(10):3194–8.
8. Leonard WJ. Cytokines and immunodeficiency diseases. Nat Rev Immunol 2001; 1:200–8.
9. Bousso P, Wahn V, Douagi I, et al. Diversity, functionality, and stability of the T cell repertoire derived in vivo from a single human T cell precursor. Proc Natl Acad Sci U S A 2000;97(1):274–8. [In Process Citation].
10. Cavazzana-Calvo M, Hacein-Bey S, De Saint Basile G, et al. Gene therapy of human severe combined immunodeficiency (SCID)-X1 disease. Science 2000; 288:669–72.
11. Gaspar HB, Parsley KL, Howe S, et al. Gene therapy of X-linked severe combined immunodeficiency by use of a pseudotyped gammaretroviral vector. Lancet 2004;364(9452):2181–7.
12. Hacein-Bey-Abina S, Le Deist F, Carlier F, et al. Sustained correction of X-linked severe combined immunodeficiency by ex vivo gene therapy. N Engl J Med 2002;346(16):1185–93.
13. Deichmann A, Hacein-Bey-Abina S, Schmidt M, et al. Vector integration is nonrandom and clustered and influences the fate of lymphopoiesis in SCID-X1 gene therapy. J Clin Invest 2007;117(8):2225–32.
14. Howe SJ, Mansour MR, Schwarzwaelder K, et al. Insertional mutagenesis combined with acquired somatic mutations causes leukemogenesis following gene therapy of SCID-X1 patients. J Clin Invest 2008;118(9):3143–50.
15. Schmidt M, Hacein-Bey-Abina S, Wissler M, et al. Clonal evidence for the transduction of CD34+ cells with lymphomyeloid differentiation potential and self-renewal capacity in the SCID-X1 gene therapy trial. Blood 2005;105(7): 2699–706.
16. Hacein-Bey-Abina S, Von Kalle C, Schmidt M, et al. LMO2-Associated clonal T cell proliferation in two patients after gene therapy for SCID-X1. Science 2003; 302(5644):415–9.
17. Hacein-Bey-Abina S, Garrigue A, Wang GP, et al. Insertional oncogenesis in 4 patients after retrovirus-mediated gene therapy of SCID-X1. J Clin Invest 2008; 118(9):3132–42.
18. Wu X, Li Y, Crise B, et al. Transcription start regions in the human genome are favored targets for MLV integration. Science 2003;300(5626):1749–51.
19. Aiuti A, Cattaneo F, Galimberti S, et al. Gene therapy for immunodeficiency due to adenosine deaminase deficiency. N Engl J Med 2009;360(5): 447–58.
20. Aiuti A, Cassani B, Andolfi G, et al. Multilineage hematopoietic reconstitution without clonal selection in ADA-SCID patients treated with stem cell gene therapy. J Clin Invest 2007;117(8):2233–40.

21. Cassani B, Montini E, Maruggi G, et al. Integration of retroviral vectors induces minor changes in the transcriptional activity of T cells from ADA-SCID patients treated with gene therapy. Blood 2009;114(17):3546–56.

22. Modlich U, Bohne J, Schmidt M, et al. Cell-culture assays reveal the importance of retroviral vector design for insertional genotoxicity. Blood 2006;108(8): 2545–53.

23. Shou Y, Ma Z, Lu T, et al. Unique risk factors for insertional mutagenesis in a mouse model of XSCID gene therapy. Proc Natl Acad Sci U S A 2006; 103(31):11730–5.

24. Montini E, Cesana D, Schmidt M, et al. Hematopoietic stem cell gene transfer in a tumor-prone mouse model uncovers low genotoxicity of lentiviral vector integration. Nat Biotechnol 2006;24(6):687–96.

25. Li CL, Xiong D, Stamatoyannopoulos G, et al. Genomic and functional assays demonstrate reduced gammaretroviral vector genotoxicity associated with use of the cHS4 chromatin insulator. Mol Ther 2009;17(4):716–24.

26. Baum C. I could die for you: new prospects for suicide in gene therapy. Mol Ther 2007;15(5):848–9.

27. Schroder AR, Shinn P, Chen H, et al. HIV-1 integration in the human genome favors active genes and local hotspots. Cell 2002;110(4):521–9.

28. Modlich U, Navarro S, Zychlinski D, et al. Insertional transformation of hematopoietic cells by self-inactivating lentiviral and gammaretroviral vectors. Mol Ther 2009;17(11):1919–28.

29. Trobridge GD, Miller DG, Jacobs MA, et al. Foamy virus vector integration sites in normal human cells. Proc Natl Acad Sci U S A 2006;103(5):1498–503.

30. Thrasher AJ, Hacein-Bey-Abina S, Gaspar HB, et al. Failure of SCID-X1 gene therapy in older patients. Blood 2005;105(11):4255–7.

31. Chinen J, Davis J, De Ravin SS, et al. Gene therapy improves immune function in preadolescents with X-linked severe combined immunodeficiency. Blood 2007; 110(1):67–73.

32. Blackburn MR, Kellems RE. Adenosine deaminase deficiency: metabolic basis of immune deficiency and pulmonary inflammation. Adv Immunol 2005;86:1–41.

33. Muul LM, Tuschong LM, Soenen SL, et al. Persistence and expression of the adenosine deaminase gene for 12 years and immune reaction to gene transfer components: long-term results of the first clinical gene therapy trial. Blood 2003;101(7):2563–9.

34. Bordignon C, Notarangelo LD, Nobili N, et al. Gene therapy in peripheral blood lymphocytes and bone marrow for ADA- immunodeficient patients. Science 1995;270(5235):470–5.

35. Kohn DB, Hershfield MS, Carbonaro D, et al. T lymphocytes with a normal ADA gene accumulate after transplantation of transduced autologous umbilical cord blood CD34+ cells in ADA-deficient SCID neonates. Nat Med 1998;4(7): 775–80.

36. Schmidt M, Carbonaro DA, Speckmann C, et al. Clonality analysis after retroviral-mediated gene transfer to CD34+ cells from the cord blood of ADA-deficient SCID neonates. Nat Med 2003;9(4):463–8.

37. Aiuti A, Slavin S, Aker M, et al. Correction of ADA-SCID by stem cell gene therapy combined with nonmyeloablative conditioning. Science 2002;296(5577):2410–3.

38. Gaspar HB, Aiuti A, Porta F, et al. How I treat ADA deficiency. Blood 2009; 114(17):3524–32.

39. Buckley RH. Molecular defects in human severe combined immunodeficiency and approaches to immune reconstitution. Annu Rev Immunol 2004;22:625–55.

40. Yates F, Malassis-Seris M, Stockholm D, et al. Gene therapy of RAG-2-/- mice: sustained correction of the immunodeficiency. Blood 2002;22:22.
41. Mostoslavsky G, Fabian AJ, Rooney S, et al. Complete correction of murine Artemis immunodeficiency by lentiviral vector-mediated gene transfer. Proc Natl Acad Sci U S A 2006;103(44):16406–11.
42. Benjelloun F, Garrigue A, Demerens-de Chappedelaine C, et al. Stable and functional lymphoid reconstitution in artemis-deficient mice following lentiviral Artemis gene transfer into hematopoietic stem cells. Mol Ther 2008;16(8):1490–9.
43. Bunting KD, Sangster MY, Ihle JN, et al. Restoration of lymphocyte function in Janus kinase 3-deficient mice by retroviral-mediated gene transfer [comments]. Nat Med 1998;4(1):58–64.
44. Adjali O, Vicente RR, Ferrand C, et al. Intrathymic administration of hematopoietic progenitor cells enhances T cell reconstitution in ZAP-70 severe combined immunodeficiency. Proc Natl Acad Sci U S A 2005;102(38):13586–91.
45. Lagresle-Peyrou C, Yates F, Malassis-Seris M, et al. Long-term immune reconstitution in RAG-1-deficient mice treated by retroviral gene therapy: a balance between efficiency and toxicity. Blood 2006;107(1):63–72.
46. Bosticardo M, Marangoni F, Aiuti A, et al. Recent advances in understanding the pathophysiology of Wiskott-Aldrich syndrome. Blood 2009;113(25):6288–95.
47. Klein C, Nguyen D, Liu CH, et al. Gene therapy for Wiskott-Aldrich syndrome: rescue of T-cell signaling and amelioration of colitis upon transplantation of retrovirally transduced hematopoietic stem cells in mice. Blood 2003;101(6): 2159–66.
48. Marangoni F, Bosticardo M, Charrier S, et al. Evidence for long-term efficacy and safety of gene therapy for Wiskott-Aldrich syndrome in preclinical models. Mol Ther 2009;17(6):1073–82.
49. Charrier S, Dupre L, Scaramuzza S, et al. Lentiviral vectors targeting WASp expression to hematopoietic cells, efficiently transduce and correct cells from WAS patients. Gene Ther 2007;14(5):415–28.
50. Dupre L, Trifari S, Follenzi A, et al. Lentiviral vector-mediated gene transfer in T cells from Wiskott-Aldrich syndrome patients leads to functional correction. Mol Ther 2004;10(5):903–15.
51. Dupre L, Marangoni F, Scaramuzza S, et al. Efficacy of gene therapy for Wiskott-Aldrich syndrome using a WAS promoter/cDNA-containing lentiviral vector and nonlethal irradiation. Hum Gene Ther 2006;17(3):303–13.
52. Boztuk K, Schmidt M, Schwaezer A, et al. HSC gene therapy in two WAS patients [abstract]. Hum Gene Ther 2009;20:1371.
53. Ozsahin H, Cavazzana-Calvo M, Notarangelo LD, et al. Long-term outcome following hematopoietic stem-cell transplantation in Wiskott-Aldrich syndrome: collaborative study of the European Society for Immunodeficiencies and European Group for Blood and Marrow Transplantation. Blood 2008;111(1):439–45.
54. Fischer A, Latour S, de Saint Basile G. Genetic defects affecting lymphocyte cytotoxicity. Curr Opin Immunol 2007;19(3):348–53.
55. Recchia A, Bonini C, Magnani Z, et al. Retroviral vector integration deregulates gene expression but has no consequence on the biology and function of transplanted T cells. Proc Natl Acad Sci U S A 2006;103(5):1457–62.
56. Ochs HD, Ziegler SF, Torgerson TR. FOXP3 acts as a rheostat of the immune response. Immunol Rev 2005;203:156–64.
57. Kerns HM, Ryu BY, Stirling BV, et al. B-cell-specific lentiviral gene therapy leads to sustained B cell functional recovery in a murine model of X-linked agammaglobulinemia. Blood 2010. [Epub ahead of print].

58. Seger RA. Modern management of chronic granulomatous disease. Br J Haematol 2008;140(3):255–66.

59. Malech HL, Maples PB, Whiting-Theobald N, et al. Prolonged production of NADPH oxidase-corrected granulocytes after gene therapy of chronic granulomatous disease. Proc Natl Acad Sci U S A 1997;94(22):12133–8.

60. Ott MG, Schmidt M, Schwarzwaelder K, et al. Correction of X-linked chronic granulomatous disease by gene therapy, augmented by insertional activation of MDS1-EVI1, PRDM16 or SETBP1. Nat Med 2006;12(4):401–9.

61. Stein S, Ott MG, Schultze-Strasser S, et al. Genomic instability and myelodysplasia with monosomy 7 consequent to EVI1 activation after gene therapy for chronic granulomatous disease. Nat Med 2010;16:198–204.

62. Kang EM, Choi U, Theobald N, et al. Retrovirus gene therapy for X-linked chronic granulomatous disease can achieve stable long-term correction of oxidase activity in peripheral blood neutrophils. Blood 2010;115(4):783–91.

63. Cartier N, Hacein-Bey-Abina S, Bartholomae CC, et al. Hematopoietic stem cell gene therapy with a lentiviral vector in X-linked adrenoleukodystrophy. Science 2009;326(5954):818–23.

64. Bauer TR Jr, Allen JM, Hai M, et al. Successful treatment of canine leukocyte adhesion deficiency by foamy virus vectors. Nat Med 2008;14(1):93–7.

65. Rottman M, Soudais C, Vogt G, et al. IFN-gamma mediates the rejection of haematopoietic stem cells in IFN-gammaR1-deficient hosts. PLoS Med 2008; 5(1):e26.

66. van Deutekom JC, Janson AA, Ginjaar IB, et al. Local dystrophin restoration with antisense oligonucleotide PRO051. N Engl J Med 2007;357(26):2677–86.

67. Porteus MH, Carroll D. Gene targeting using zinc finger nucleases. Nat Biotechnol 2005;23(8):967–73.

68. Redondo P, Prieto J, Munoz IG, et al. Molecular basis of xeroderma pigmentosum group C DNA recognition by engineered meganucleases. Nature 2008; 456(7218):107–11.

69. Urnov FD, Miller JC, Lee YL, et al. Highly efficient endogenous human gene correction using designed zinc-finger nucleases. Nature 2005;435(7042):646–51.

# Gene Therapy for Adenosine Deaminase Deficiency

Barbara Cappelli, MD[a,b], Alessandro Aiuti, MD, PhD[a,b,c],*

KEYWORDS

- Immune deficiency • Adenosine deaminase
- Gene therapy • Haematopoietic stem cell
- Reduced-intensity conditioning regimen

Primary immunodeficiency diseases (PIDs) are a genetically heterogeneous group of inherited disorders that affect distinct components of the innate and adaptive immune system, with impairment of their differentiation and/or functions.[1,2] Severe combined immunodeficiencies (SCIDs) represent about 15% of PIDs, ranging between 1:75,000 and 1:100,000 live births.[3] Adenosine deaminase (ADA) deficiency is a rare autosomal recessive disease belonging to the SCID group[4,5] (OMIM#102700). ADA deficiency represents the cause of approximately 10% to 20% of all cases of SCIDs,[4,6,7] with an overall prevalence in Europe that can be estimated to range between 1:375,000 and 1:660,000 live births, equivalent to 0.026 to 0.015 every 10,000 live births. Since 1972, ADA-SCID became the first immunodeficiency for which a specific molecular defect was identified, at both genetic and biochemical level.[8] ADA is a ubiquitous intracellular enzyme of purine metabolism. It catalyzes the irreversible deamination of adenosine (Ado) and deoxyadenosine (dAdo) in the purine catabolic pathway. Its deficiency results in metabolic toxicity because of the impairment of purine metabolism that leads to the intracellular accumulation of metabolic substrates, deoxyadenosine-X-phosphate (dAXP) and Ado. These metabolites are highly toxic for the cells, especially for lymphocytes and their precursors.[6] The human ADA gene is located on the long arm of chromosome 20 (20q12-q3.11).[7] Mutations in the ADA gene cause alterations in enzyme's activity, stability, and survival, leading to accumulation of Ado, dAdo, and adenine deoxyribonucleotides (dAXP) in plasma, red blood cells, and

[a] San Raffaele Telethon Institute for Gene Therapy (HSR-TIGET), San Raffaele Scientific Institute, via Olgettina 58, Milan 20132, Italy
[b] Pediatric Immunohematology and Bone Marrow Transplantation Unit, San Raffaele Scientific Institute, via Olgettina 60, Milan 20132, Italy
[c] Department of Pediatrics, Children's Hospital Bambino Gesù, University of Rome Tor Vergata, P.zza S. Onofrio, Rome 4- 00165, Italy
* Corresponding author. San Raffaele Telethon Institute for Gene Therapy (HSR-TIGET), San Raffaele Scientific Institute, via Olgettina 58, Milan 20132, Italy.
E-mail address: a.aiuti@hsr.it

Immunol Allergy Clin N Am 30 (2010) 249–260
doi:10.1016/j.iac.2010.02.003
0889-8561/10/$ – see front matter © 2010 Elsevier Inc. All rights reserved.

tissues. About 70 known different mutations have been identified in the ADA gene.[7,9,10] The main features of the disease are impaired differentiation and functions of T, B, and natural killer (NK) cells; recurrent infections; and failure to thrive. In addition, nonimmunologic abnormalities occur as the consequence of the systemic metabolic defect as a result of the accumulation of purine toxic metabolites.[4,5,11] Similar to other SCIDs, ADA-SCID is a fatal disease that usually leads to death in the first year of life, if not treated. However, among the SCIDs, it is one of the most difficult to handle clinically because of the concomitant systemic metabolic toxicity, which is typical of the disease (**Fig. 1**).

At present, the different therapeutic options available for its treatment are hematopoietic stem cell transplantation (HSCT), enzyme replacement therapy (ERT) with polyethylene glycol–modified ADA (PEG-ADA), and gene therapy (GT).

## HEMATOPOIETIC STEM CELL TRANSPLANTATION

HSCTs for ADA-SCID represent about 11% of total transplants for SCID performed in Europe.[12] HSCT from an HLA-identical family donor is the gold standard treatment for patients with ADA-SCID, but it is available only for a minority of patients.[12] When feasible, this therapeutic procedure has a favorable outcome, with an overall 3-year survival of 81% in the European Society for Immunodeficiencies registry, with most recent transplant survival rates exceeding 90%, if HSCTs are performed promptly.[13–15] An overview of patients with ADA-SCID recruited in European and North American centers showed after matched sibling and matched family donor

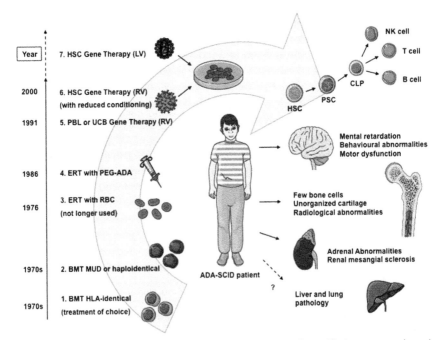

**Fig. 1.** Development of therapeutic options in ADA-SCID and specific immune and nonimmune features of the disease. (*From* Sauer AV, Aiuti A. New insights into the pathogenesis of adenosine deaminase-severe combined immunodeficiency and progress in gene therapy. Curr Opin Allergy Clin Immunol 2009;9(6):496–502; with permission.)

(often available due to the high incidence of consanguineous pedigrees) HSCTs an overall 1-year survival of 87% and 88%, respectively.[15] This type of HSCT is usually given without conditioning to reduce the risk of chemotherapy-associated toxicity. It usually results in a split chimerism, with only T lymphocytes of donor origin and other lineages, including B cells, remaining of host origin.[12,16] This may lead to variable correction of B-cell deficiency and of the metabolic defect.[16] In fact, dAdo purine metabolites, even if dramatically reduced compared with untreated patients, remain often higher than normal values (average dATP, 100 nmol/mL),[17] and plasma levels of Ado are persistently high, apparently without adverse effects. In addition, several cases in which neurologic complications of ADA-SCID are not corrected by the transplant have been described.[18]

## HSCT FROM UNRELATED AND ALTERNATIVE DONORS

Transplants from matched unrelated donors (MUDs) or from umbilical cord blood (UCB) have been introduced in the past years as potential options for ADA-SCIDs. These transplants require typically chemotherapy and immunosuppressive drugs to accomplish complete donor chimerism in all cell lineages and long-term immune reconstitution. The ideal conditioning regimen has not been defined yet, with different groups using different approaches. Bone marrow or mobilized peripheral blood donors are searched worldwide in the bone marrow registries, but only less than 50% of the patients will find a fully matched donor. UCB units are readily available, and the degree of matching is less strict, being based on 6 alleles only (HLA-A, -B, -DR). However, so far, there is little available information on the outcome of MUD or UCB transplants for ADA-SCID in Europe. Recently, Gaspar and colleagues[15] showed a survival of 67% after fully matched unrelated donor transplants. Moreover, surviving MUD HSCT patients showed neurologic disturbances and late onset behavioral problems with developmental delay, typical of patients with ADA-SCID.[18,19] Cumulative data from unrelated UCB transplants in patients with primary immunodeficiencies showed a 5-year survival rate of 70%,[20] and all surviving patients presented complete immunologic reconstitution, but data on UCB transplants in patients with ADA-SCID are very limited.[15]

In conclusion, in the absence of an HLA-identical family donor, bone marrow transplantation for patients with ADA-SCID remains a treatment with a high risk of death. This is mainly because of a significant treatment-related toxicity, especially in MUD HSCT performed with conventional conditioning.

As an alternative source, child's parents' HSCs have also been used with the advantage that a donor is always and immediately available. However, this procedure is associated with many drawbacks, such as the increased risk of rejection and graft-versus-host disease (GVHD) or infections (due to the need of T-cell depletion). Data from a recent review show after mismatched unrelated and mismatched family donor transplants (mainly haploidentical) a survival of only 29% and 43% respectively, with most deaths in the first few months after transplant.[15]

Because of the encouraging experience in other forms of SCID, the Duke Center, USA, has pursued HSCT from T-cell–depleted parental bone marrow early in life and without conditioning to avoid toxicity of high-dose chemotherapy.[21] However, in ADA-SCID, this type of transplant is less effective than in other forms of SCID, with only 7 of 19 patients treated achieving engraftment of donor T lymphocytes.[15]

## ENZYME REPLACEMENT THERAPY

ERT was introduced for the first time as lifesaving, noncurative treatment in 1986 for patients lacking an HLA-compatible donor.[22,23] The rationale for ERT is based on the concept that maintaining high ADA activity in plasma, a weekly or twice-weekly intramuscular injection of PEG-ADA, eliminates Ado and dAdo derived from nucleotide and nucleic acid turnover. This protects immature lymphoid cells from apoptosis triggered by dAdo-induced dATP pool expansion, and from other mechanisms, restoring protective immune function in most patients in approximately 2 to 4 months.[23] Systemic ERT may also prevent metabolic toxicity to other organs, which may cause hepatic and neurologic dysfunction in some ADA-deficient patients. At present, updated data on 185 patients treated with PEG-ADA through September 2008 have been collected.[15] Approximately 20% of patients had died while on therapy, whereas 20% and 8% had discontinued ERT to undergo a potentially curative procedure such as HSCT and GT, respectively. Half of the deaths on ERT occurred within the first 6 months (40% in the first month), resulting from conditions present at diagnosis. The overall probability of surviving 20 years on ERT is estimated to be 78%. A patient alive 6 months after starting ERT had approximately 90% probability of surviving the next 12 years. Life-threatening adverse effects of ERT include refractory hemolytic anemia, chronic pulmonary insufficiency, and lymphoproliferative disorders and, rarely, hepatocellular carcinoma and infections.[5,15,23] Moreover, there is general agreement about the inadequacy of the immunologic reconstitution produced by PEG-ADA in a large fraction of patients on the long term (10–15 years). This is, at present, its biggest limitation.

## GENE THERAPY

In the last decade, experimental GT approaches have been developed as successful alternative strategies.[24–26] Current GT approaches are based on the insertion of a healthy copy of the ADA gene into HSCs, although in the initial studies mature lymphocytes were also used as target cells. The ADA complementary DNA is transferred to the cells by the use of viral vectors that stably integrate into the human genome and transmit the therapeutic gene to the progeny of HSCs. The rational for GT resides on several potential advantages over ERT and HSCT.[25] Because it is an autologous procedure, transplantation of gene-corrected HSCs is potentially applicable to all patients, independent from the availability of a donor, with no delay for donor search. Moreover, the use of autologous gene-corrected stem cells avoids rejection and GVHD because of HLA mismatches or minor antigen incompatibility. Finally, GT does not require the use of immunosuppressive prophylaxes or high-dose conditioning regimens associated with organ toxicity (liver, lung, kidney, central nervous system), prolonged period of myelosuppression, and increased risks of infections.

Moreover, GT may be sufficient to definitively treat a patient, thus avoiding the need for lifelong ERT supplementation and its high burden in terms of costs and patients' quality of life. Furthermore, there are several evidence from preclinical and clinical observations that intracellular ADA delivered by engineered HSC or healthy donor transplant is more effective than exogenously administered ADA by ERT.[27]

Several clinical studies have investigated the safety and efficacy of ADA gene transfer into autologous hematopoietic cells using retroviral vectors. In the initial trials, 19 patients received infusions of transduced lymphocytes or hematopoietic progenitor cells.[27–33] No toxicity was observed, and in most patients, transduced T cells persisted in the circulation several years after infusion. However, the low gene transfer efficiency and engraftment levels observed in these patients did not allow to achieve a significant correction of the immunologic and metabolic defects, and all patients continued ERT.

However, this substitutive treatment might have abolished the selective growth advantage for gene-corrected cells. This hypothesis was confirmed by the observation of the case of 1 patient who discontinued PEG-ADA after showing inadequate immune reconstitution after ERT and repeated infusion of gene-corrected mature lymphocytes.[31] After ERT withdrawal, T cells containing the normal ADA gene progressively replaced the untransduced cells, resulting in restoration of normal T-cell functions and antibody responses to neoantigen. However, infusion of mature T cells was not sufficient to allow full correction of the metabolic defect, likely because of the limited mass of detoxifying cells.[31]

### Rationale for Patients' Conditioning in Gene Therapy

Nonmyeloablative conditioning for patients with SCID undergoing allogeneic HSCT has shown that mainly T-lymphocyte line cells of the healthy donor engraft long term, whereas most or all B-lymphoid line cells usually do not engraft, and the other hematopoietic (myeloid, erythroid) lines remain those of the host. Also, the recent results obtained by the authors' group[26,34] and other researchers with SCID GT[32,33] indicate that in the absence of myeloablative therapy, engineered progenitors of T lymphocytes and mature T lymphocytes carry a selective advantage for growth that enables them to prevail over-diseased, nontransduced cells. However, engraftment levels of engineered B-lymphoid line cells and other hematopoietic cells are very low and do not reach therapeutic levels. This could be attributed to the presence of resident progenitor cells (B cells, myeloid cells, HSCs) competing in the bone marrow niche.

In particular, the experience throughout the years with GT of ADA-SCID has highlighted the potential and limitations of reconstitution limited to the T-cell lineage. On the other hand, the accumulation of toxic metabolites of ADA in lymphoid organs inhibits the development and growth not only of T lymphocytes but also of B lymphocytes, suggesting that, at the level of differentiating cells, gene-corrected cells within the B-cell lineage should carry a selective advantage once progenitors have engrafted. Furthermore, there is indirect evidence that the presence of particularly high levels of these metabolites could damage nonlymphoid organs also. The degree of metabolic control that can be achieved by the mass of cells able to produce the ADA gene and the correction of the defect of the B-lymphoid line and of the other hematopoietic lines are therefore the critical factors for the success of the approach based on GT. Thus, chemotherapeutic conditioning before transplanting engineered HSCs could be a key factor for a complete and persistent success of ADA-SCID GT by allowing the engraftment of multipotent progenitors.

A second objective of chemotherapeutic conditioning is to remove the ADA defective cells, when they are responsible for concomitant disorders such as autoimmune manifestations.

### HEMATOPOIETIC STEM CELL GENE THERAPY

Autologous HSCs have been considered the optimal target cells for long-term, full correction of the ADA-SCID defect. In the past 10 years, more than 30 infants with ADA deficiency have been treated using retroviral vectors in Italy (The San Raffaele Telethon Institute for Gene Therapy, Milano), United Kingdom (Great Ormond Street Hospital, London), United States of America (Childrens Hospital of Los Angeles [CHLA]–National Institutes of Health [NIH]), and Japan (Hokkaido University, Sapporo).[26,33–37] Number of treated patients per center and type of vector and conditioning regimen used are shown in **Table 1**. Results on the first 10 patients treated in Milano have been recently reported.[26] Patients received, after a busulfan-based conditioning

**Table 1**
**Clinical trials of hematopoietic stem cell gene therapy for ADA-SCID conducted in the last decade**

| Study | No of Patients Treated | Retroviral Vector | Conditioning Regimen | PEG-ADA Discontinuation (Yes/No) |
|---|---|---|---|---|
| HSR-TIGET[26,34] | 15 | GIADAI | Busulfan (4 mg/kg) | Yes |
| GOSH[15,17] | 5 | SFFV-ADA-WPRE | Melphalan (140 mg/m$^2$) | Yes |
| CHLA-NIH 1[33,35] | 4 | GCsap-M-ADA and MND-ADA | No | No |
| CHLA-NIH 2[33,35] | 6 | GCsap-M-ADA and MND-ADA | Busulfan (75–90 mg/m$^2$) | Yes |
| Hokkaido[36] | 2 | GCsap-M-ADA | No | Yes |

*Abbreviations:* HSR-TIGET, The San Raffaele Telethon Institute for Gene Therapy, Milano, Italy; MND, myeloproliferative sarcoma virus [MPSV] enhancer, negative control region deleted, dl587rev primer binding site substituted; SFFV, spleen focus-forming virus.

protocol (4 mg/kg i.v.), a high dose of CD34$^+$ cells (mean $8.2 \times 10^6$ CD34$^+$ cells/kg), containing an average of 28.6% of transduced progenitors. Levels of transduction were similar to those of other studies, but the large number of CD34$^+$ cells infused in most patients may have been important for the success of this study. High levels of gene marking were seen in peripheral T (88% average marking), B (52%), and NK (59%) cells (**Fig. 2**). Moreover, the detection in peripheral blood and bone marrow of ADA-transduced cells in multiple lineages (myeloid, erythroid, megakaryocytic) demonstrated the efficacy of the reduced-intensity conditioning regimen in achieving substantial HSC engraftment (see **Fig. 2**). Nine patients have benefited from GT, showing effective adequate systemic detoxification, reduction in the frequency of infection, and improvement of their weight-height growth curve. Moreover, a progressive reconstitution of T-cell counts and functions was also observed, although at slower rate with respect to standard HSCT.[26] Five patients showed complete immune reconstitution with discontinuation of intravenous immunoglobulin and humoral immune responses to vaccinal and microbial antigens (**Fig. 3**). On the other hand, 1 patient who experienced autoimmunity during ERT showed an insufficient engraftment and, because of the recurrency of autoimmunity, continued to require steroid treatment.[26]

Five additional patients have been treated with promising results. At present, all 15 patients treated with this protocol are alive, and only 2 patients have required ERT after GT.[37]

In a similar trial performed in London using an alternative retroviral construct (viral spleen focus-forming virus–long terminal repeat promoter for ADA gene transcription) and a single-dose melphalan conditioning regimen, 5 patients have been treated (see **Table 1**).[15,17] Of the 5 treated patients, 2 have shown very good immune reconstitution and are clinically well, 1 patient restarted PEG-ADA, and 2 patients failed GT because of a poor stem cell harvest and a low-level stem cell transduction efficiency, respectively. In the 2 most successfully reconstituted patients, ADA expression was observed in different hematopoietic lineages, including red blood cells, leading to effective metabolic control. In both patients, recovery of thymopoiesis was demonstrated after GT. Gene correction was proved in most T cells and NK cells, whereas significant gene marking was also observed in granulocytes and monocytes.

Encouraging results have also been recently reported in similar studies performed at the NIH and CHLA (see **Table 1**).[15,35] In a first study, 4 patients received GT without

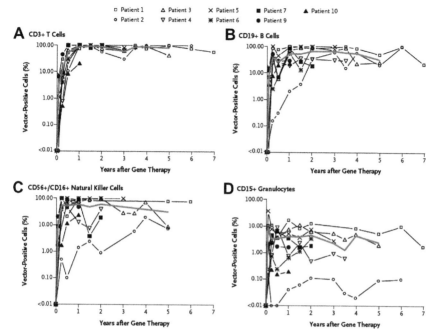

**Fig. 2.** Persistence of ADA-transduced cells in different lineages after gene therapy. The proportions of vector-positive cells (on a log10 scale) for 9 patients with ADA-SCID treated with gene therapy and on average (*red line*) are shown for different cell lineages from peripheral blood samples: $CD3^+$ T cells (panel *A*), $CD19^+$ B cells (panel *B*), $CD56^+/CD16^+$ NK cells (panel *C*), and $CD15^+$ granulocytes (panel *D*). (*From* Aiuti A, Cattaneo F, Galimberti S, et al. Gene therapy for immunodeficiency due to adenosine deaminase deficiency. N Engl J Med 2009;360(5):447–58; with permission.)

conditioning, leading to low levels of engraftment and no sustained immunologic improvement while continuing ERT.[33] In a second clinical trial, 6 patients were treated with low-dose busulfan in combination with PEG-ADA withdrawal. Two patients with a follow-up longer than 1 year showed a normalization of in vitro T-cell function and improvement of immunoglobulin production, in 1 case associated to normal responses to vaccines. In all but 1 case, production of ADA by peripheral blood mononuclear cells resulted in sustained detoxification of purine metabolites at levels comparable to those observed after HSCT.[15] One patient with a pre-GT cytogenetic abnormality experienced a prolonged cytopenia after busulfan conditioning.[15]

An alternative GT strategy based on PEG-ADA withdrawal without myeloablative conditioning was attempted on 2 patients with ADA-SCID in Japan. Preliminary reports have shown some degree of immunologic reconstitution, at lower level than in patients pretreated with conditioning, but a longer follow-up is required for full evaluation of this approach (see **Table 1**).[36]

All together, these results showed the efficacy of infusion of autologous ADA gene–corrected HSCs in combination with a reduced-intensity conditioning regimen.

## SAFETY OF ADA-SCID GENE THERAPY

A potential risk associated with gene transfer can be represented by "insertional oncogenesis," by which a retroviral vector may land into the genome adjacent to cellular genes, such as proto-oncogene, leading to inappropriate expression of the

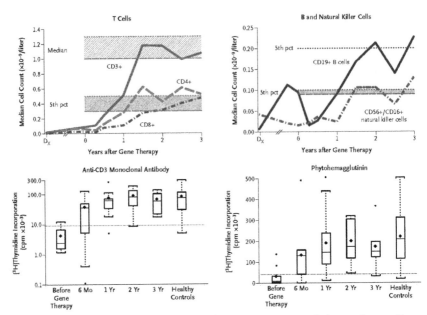

**Fig. 3.** Immune reconstitution after gene therapy. Upper panel shows the median cell counts for CD3[+] T cells, CD4[+] T cells, and CD8[+] T cells (*left*) and B cells and NK cells (*right*) after gene therapy. Reference values for age are also shown as shaded areas or dotted lines.[26] Bottom panel shows data for the in vitro proliferative responses to anti-CD3 monoclonal antibody (on a log10 scale, *left side*) and to phytohemagglutinin (on a linear scale, *right side*). The data are expressed as counts per minute (cpm) in ADA-deficient patients and in healthy controls. The dashed horizontal line represents the 5th percentile for healthy controls. (*From* Aiuti A, Cattaneo F, Galimberti S, et al. Gene therapy for immunodeficiency due to ADA deficiency. N Engl J Med 2009;360(5):447–58; with permission.)

neighboring gene. This event may lead to clonal proliferation and eventually leukemic proliferation, as observed in 5 patients with SCID-X1 who developed a T-cell leukemia and 2 patients with chronic granulomatous disease who manifested with myelodysplasia due to monosomy 7, 31 to 68 months after GT.[38,39]

However, in addition to vector-mediated activation of cellular genes, it is believed that other factors including the disease background, the nature of the transgene, and the acquisition of other genetic abnormalities unrelated to vector insertions are also needed for aberrant expansion. So far, the cumulative experience of GT for ADA-SCID did not reveal the occurrence of clonal expansion or leukemic proliferation, indicating that it has a favorable risk-benefit profile. This is in agreement with the finding of a polyclonal pattern of T-cell receptor repertoire and vector integrations in treated patients.[26,40]

Moreover, in vitro studies on transduced clones generated ex vivo from patients with ADA-SCID, several years after GT, failed to show significant signs of perturbation of neighboring genes and did not lead to growth advantage or alteration in cellular behavior.[40]

## PERSPECTIVES FOR NOVEL GENE TRANSFER APPROACHES

For future applications in the context of ADA-SCID and other inherited primary immunodeficiencies, the use of self-inactivating human immunodeficiency virus

(HIV)–derived lentiviral vectors may improve the safety and efficacy of gene transfer into HSCs. These vectors offer a unique combination of advantages over retroviral vectors because they integrate efficiently into HSCs, allow stable and robust transgene expression, and significantly alleviate the safety concerns associated with retroviral vector integration. In addition, they can be adapted to contain physiologic cellular promoters rather than viral promoters used for retroviral vectors. Lentiviral vectors have recently entered the clinic with wide-ranging applications, as several trials are ongoing or are beginning in Europe and the United States to treat HIV infection,[41] neurodegenerative syndromes,[42] primary immunodeficiencies,[43] or genetic diseases such as thalassemia.

The efficacy of lentiviral vector–mediated ADA gene transfer has been recently explored in preclinical mouse models of ADA deficiency using 2 different strategies. In the first approach, murine HSCs transduced with lentiviral vectors transplanted into ADA-deficient mice resulted in full metabolic detoxification, restoration of ADA activity, and differentiation and immune functions of lymphoid cells.[44] Pretransplant irradiation was crucial for long-term survival of ADA−/− mice because animals receiving transplants without irradiation died 2 weeks after transplantation due to poor engraftment. In a different approach, a SIN–lentiviral vector was used to treat neonatal ADA−/− mice directly by intravenous injection.[45] In addition to prolonged survival, mice showed significantly increased lymphoid cell counts and reconstitution of T-cell proliferation, although no selective advantage of gene-corrected T cells was observed.

Alternative GT approaches based on sophisticated system that allow gene correction or gene editing[46,47] could represent a further improvement in safety over integrating vectors, but their clinical application requires further optimization and testing at preclinical level.

## SUMMARY

In the last decade, GT has been developed as a successful alternative strategy for patients affected by ADA-SCID lacking an HLA-identical sibling donor. This approach has been shown to be well tolerated and efficacious. The introduction of a reduced-intensity conditioning regimen has been identified as a crucial factor in achieving adequate engraftment of HSCs and therapeutic levels of ADA. The future development of novel vector technology, such as lentiviral vectors, might provide a superior efficacy and safety profile. The prospects for extending the application of GT to a broader spectrum of genetic diseases, including primary immune deficiencies, remain strong.

## ACKNOWLEDGMENTS

This work was supported by Fondazione Telethon.

## REFERENCES

1. Rosen FS, Cooper MD, Wedgwood RJ. The primary immunodeficiencies. N Engl J Med 1995;333(7):431–40.
2. Geha RS, Notarangelo LD, Casanova JL, et al. Primary immunodeficiency diseases: an update from the International Union of Immunological Societies Primary Immunodeficiency Diseases Classification Committee. J Allergy Clin Immunol 2007;120(4):776–94.
3. Fischer A, Cavazzana-Calvo M, De Saint Basile G, et al. Naturally occurring primary deficiencies of the immune system. Annu Rev Immunol 1997;15:93–124.

4. Hirschorn R, Candotti F. Immunodeficiency due to defects of purine metabolism. In: Ochs H, Smith C, Puck J, editors. Primary immunodeficiency diseases. Oxford (UK): Oxford University Press; 2006. p. 169–96.
5. Sauer AV, Aiuti A. New insights into the pathogenesis of adenosine deaminase-severe combined immunodeficiency and progress in gene therapy. Curr Opin Allergy Clin Immunol 2009;9(6):496–502.
6. Cassani B, Mirolo M, Cattaneo F, et al. Altered intracellular and extracellular signaling leads to impaired T-cell functions in ADA-SCID patients. Blood 2008; 111(8):4209–19.
7. Valerio D, Duyvesteyn MG, Dekker BM, et al. Adenosine deaminase: characterization and expression of a gene with a remarkable promoter. EMBO J 1985; 4(2):437–43.
8. Giblett ER, Anderson JE, Cohen F, et al. Adenosine deaminase deficiency in two patients with severely impaired cellular immunity. Lancet 1972;2(7786):1067–9.
9. Arredondo-Vega FX, Santisteban I, Daniels S, et al. Adenosine deaminase deficiency: genotype-phenotype correlations based on expressed activity of 29 mutant alleles. Am J Hum Genet 1998;63(4):1049–59.
10. Hirschhorn R, Tzall S, Ellenbogen A. Hot spot mutations in adenosine deaminase deficiency. Proc Natl Acad Sci U S A 1990;87(16):6171–5.
11. Booth C, Hershfield M, Notarangelo L, et al. Management options for adenosine deaminase deficiency; proceedings of the EBMT satellite workshop (Hamburg, March 2006). Clin Immunol (Orlando, Fla) 2007;123(2):139–47.
12. Antoine C, Muller S, Cant A, et al. Long-term survival and transplantation of haemopoietic stem cells for immunodeficiencies: report of the European experience 1968–99. Lancet 2003;361(9357):553–60.
13. Buckley RH, Schiff SE, Schiff RI, et al. Hematopoietic stem-cell transplantation for the treatment of severe combined immunodeficiency. N Engl J Med 1999;340(7): 508–16.
14. Grunebaum E, Mazzolari E, Porta F, et al. Bone marrow transplantation for severe combined immune deficiency. JAMA 2006;295(5):508–18.
15. Gaspar HB, Aiuti A, Porta F, et al. How I treat ADA deficiency. Blood 2009; 114(17):3524–32.
16. Hirschhorn R, Roegner MV, Kuritsky L, et al. Bone marrow transplantation only partially restores purine metabolites to normal in adenosine deaminase-deficient patients. J Clin Invest 1981;68(6):1387–93.
17. Gaspar HB, Bjorkegren E, Parsley K, et al. Successful reconstitution of immunity in ADA-SCID by stem cell gene therapy following cessation of PEG-ADA and use of mild reconditioning. Mol Ther 2006;14(4):505–13.
18. Rogers MH, Lwin R, Fairbanks L, et al. Cognitive and behavioral abnormalities in adenosine deaminase deficient severe combined immunodeficiency. J Pediatr 2001;139(1):44–50.
19. Honig M, Albert MH, Schulz A, et al. Patients with adenosine deaminase deficiency surviving after hematopoietic stem cell transplantation are at high risk of CNS complications. Blood 2007;109(8):3595–602.
20. Diaz de Heredia C, Ortega JJ, Diaz MA, et al. Unrelated cord blood transplantation for severe combined immunodeficiency and other primary immunodeficiencies. Bone Marrow Transplant 2008;41(7):627–33.
21. Railey MD, Lokhnygina Y, Buckley RH. Long-term clinical outcome of patients with severe combined immunodeficiency who received related donor bone marrow transplants without pretransplant chemotherapy or post-transplant GVHD prophylaxis. J Pediatr 2009;155(6):834–40.

22. Hershfield MS, Buckley RH, Greenberg ML, et al. Treatment of adenosine deaminase deficiency with polyethylene glycol-modified adenosine deaminase. N Engl J Med 1987;316(10):589–96.
23. Hershfield MS. PEG-ADA replacement therapy for adenosine deaminase deficiency: an update after 8.5 years. Clin Immunol Immunopathol 1995;76(3 Pt 2): S228–32.
24. Thrasher AJ. Gene therapy for primary immunodeficiencies. Immunol Allergy Clin North Am 2008;28(2):457–71.
25. Kohn DB, Candotti F. Gene therapy fulfilling its promise. N Engl J Med 2009; 360(5):518–21.
26. Aiuti A, Cattaneo F, Galimberti S, et al. Gene therapy for immunodeficiency due to adenosine deaminase deficiency. N Engl J Med 2009;360(5):447–58.
27. Aiuti A, Ficara F, Cattaneo F, et al. Gene therapy for adenosine deaminase deficiency. Curr Opin Allergy Clin Immunol 2003;3(6):461–6.
28. Kohn DB, Hershfield MS, Carbonaro D, et al. T lymphocytes with a normal ADA gene accumulate after transplantation of transduced autologous umbilical cord blood CD34+ cells in ADA-deficient SCID neonates. Nat Med 1998;4(7):775–80.
29. Blaese RM, Culver KW, Miller AD, et al. T lymphocyte-directed gene therapy for ADA- SCID: initial trial results after 4 years. Science 1995;270(5235):475–80.
30. Bordignon C, Notarangelo LD, Nobili N, et al. Gene therapy in peripheral blood lymphocytes and bone marrow for ADA- immunodeficient patients. Science 1995;270:470–5.
31. Aiuti A, Vai S, Mortellaro A, et al. Immune reconstitution in ADA-SCID after PBL gene therapy and discontinuation of enzyme replacement. Nat Med 2002;8(5): 423–5.
32. Cavazzana-Calvo M, Hacein BS, de Saint Basile G, et al. Gene therapy of human severe combined immunodeficiency (SCID)-X1 disease. Science 2000;288(5466): 669–72.
33. Sokolic R, Kesserwan C, Candotti F. Recent advances in gene therapy for severe congenital immunodeficiency diseases. Curr Opin Hematol 2008;15:375–80.
34. Aiuti A, Slavin S, Aker M, et al. Correction of ADA-SCID by stem cell gene therapy combined with nonmyeloablative conditioning. Science 2002;296:2410–3.
35. Engel BC, Podsakoff GM, Ireland JL, et al. Prolonged pancytopenia in a gene therapy patient with ADA-deficient SCID and trisomy 8 mosaicism: a case report. Blood 2007;109(2):503–6.
36. Otsu M, Nakajima M, Kida M, et al. Stem cell gene therapy with no pre-conditioning for the ADA-deficiency patients leads to generalized detoxification and delayed, but steady hematological reconstitution [abstract]. Mol Ther 2006;13:S418.
37. Aiuti A, Roncarolo MG. Ten years of gene therapy for primary immunedeficiencies. Hematology Am Soc Hematol Educ Program 2009:682–9.
38. Hacein-Bey-Abina S, Von Kalle C, Schmidt M, et al. LMO2-associated clonal cell proliferation in two patients after gene therapy for SCID-X1. Science 2003; 302(5644):415–9.
39. Stein S, Ott MG, Schultze-Strasser S, et al. Genomic instability and myelodysplasia with monosomy 7 consequent to EVI1 activation after gene therapy for chronic granulomatous disease. Nat Med 2010;16(2):198–204.
40. Aiuti A, Cassani B, Andolfi G, et al. Multilineage hematopoietic reconstitution without clonal selection in ADA-SCID patients treated with stem cell gene therapy. J Clin Invest 2007;117(8):2233–40.
41. Rossi JJ, June CH, Kohn DB. Genetic therapies against HIV [review]. Nat Biotechnol 2007;25(12):1444–54.

42. Cartier N, Hacein-Bey-Abina S, Bartholomae CC, et al. Hematopoietic stem cell gene therapy with a lentiviral vector in X-linked adrenoleukodystrophy. Science 2009;326(5954):818–23.
43. Marangoni F, Bosticardo M, Charrier S, et al. Evidence for long-term efficacy and safety of gene therapy for Wiskott-Aldrich syndrome in preclinical models. Mol Ther 2009;17(6):1073–82.
44. Mortellaro A, Hernandez RJ, Guerrini MM, et al. Ex vivo gene therapy with lentiviral vectors rescues adenosine deaminase (ADA)-deficient mice and corrects their immune and metabolic defects. Blood 2006;108(9):2979–88.
45. Carbonaro DA, Jin X, Petersen D, et al. In vivo transduction by intravenous injection of a lentiviral vector expressing human ADA into neonatal ADA gene knockout mice: a novel form of enzyme replacement therapy for ADA deficiency. Mol Ther 2006;13(6):1110–20.
46. Urnov FD, Miller JC, Lee YL, et al. Highly efficient endogenous human gene correction using designed zinc-finger nucleases. Nature 2005;435(7042):646–51.
47. Lombardo A, Genovese P, Beausejour CM, et al. Gene editing in human stem cells using zinc finger nucleases and integrase-defective lentiviral vector delivery. Nat Biotechnol 2007;25(11):1298–306.

# Indications for Hemopoietic Stem Cell Transplantation

Chaim M. Roifman, MD, FRCPC, FCACB[a],*, Alain Fischer, MD, PhD[b,c,d],
Luigi D. Notarangelo, MD[e], M. Teresa de la Morena, MD[f],
Reinhard A. Seger, MD[g]

---

**KEYWORDS**

- Hemopoietic stem cell transplantation
- Primary immunodeficiency • T cell defects
- Autoimmune syndromes

---

The following is a complete list of definite as well as possible indications for hemopoietic stem cell transplantation in primary immunodeficiency (limitations are provided as footnotes).

1. Severe combined immunodeficiency (SCID)
   Caused by mutations in:
   ARTEMIS
   $CD3\delta,\varepsilon,\zeta$
   CD45
   $IL2R\gamma$
   $IL7R\alpha$
   Jak-3
   RAG1/RAG2
   Adenylate kinase-2 gene (AK2)
   Adenosine deaminase (ADA) deficiency[1,2]
   Unknown genotype

---

[a] Division of Immunology & Allergy, The Canadian Centre for Primary Immunodeficiency, The Jeffrey Modell Research Laboratory for the Diagnosis of Primary Immunodeficiency, The Hospital for Sick Children, University of Toronto, 555 University Avenue, Toronto, ON M5G 1X8, Canada

[b] University Paris Descartes, Necker Medical School, Paris 75015, France

[c] Institut National de la Santé et de la Recherche Médicale, U768, Necker Hospital, 149 rue de Sèrves, Paris 75015, France

[d] Unité d'Immuno-Hématologie Pédiatrique, Necker Hospital, Assistance Publique-Hôpitaux de Paris, 149 rue de Sèvres, Paris 75015, France

[e] Division of Immunology, and Manton Center for Orphan Disease Research, Children's Hospital, Harvard Medical School, Boston, MA 02115, USA

[f] Division of Allergy and Immunology, University of Texas Southwestern Medical Center at Dallas, 5323 Harry Hines Boulevard, Dallas, TX 75390-9063, USA

[g] Division Immunology/Haematology, University Children's Hospital of Zurich, Zurich, Switzerland

* Corresponding author.

*E-mail address:* chaim.roifman@sickkids.ca

[1] MRD-BMT only.

[2] Limited to infancy and childhood; or severe form, if evidence on adults is lacking.

Immunol Allergy Clin N Am 30 (2010) 261–262
doi:10.1016/j.iac.2010.03.004
0889-8561/10/$ – see front matter © 2010 Elsevier Inc. All rights reserved.

**immunology.theclinics.com**

2. Profound T cell defects (CID)[2,3]
   - Caused by mutation in:
     IL2Rα
     Orai-1
     Zap-70
     CD3γ
     CD40L deficiency[1,2,3]
     Major histocompatibility antigens (MHC) class II deficiency
     Unknown genotype
     Omenn syndrome Caused by mutation in:
     RAG1/2
     RMRP
     DNA ligase IV
     ADA
     IL7Rα
     Unknown genotype
   - Profound T cell defects associated with metabolic or multiorgan syndromes
     Cartilage hair hypoplasia (CHH)[2,3]
     Cernunnos deficiency
     DNA ligase 4 deficiency[2,3,4]
     Purine nucleoside phosphorylase (PNP) deficiency
     Wiskott-Aldrich syndrome (WAS)[2,3]
     Dyskeratosis congenita (Hoyeraal-Hreidarsson syndrome)[4]
     NF-Kappa-B Essential Modulator (NEMO) deficiency[4]
     Schimke syndrome[2,3,4]
     STIM1 deficiency
3. Autoimmune and autoinflammatory syndromes
   Autoimmune lymphoproliferative syndrome (ALPS)[2,3]
   Immune dysregulation, polyendocrinopathy, enteropathy, and X-linked inheri-
     tance (IPEX)[2,3]
   IL10R deficiency
   Mevalonate deficiency
4. Innate immune defects
   Chronic granulomatous disease[2,3]
   IFN-γR deficiency[2,4]
   Leukocyte adhesion deficiency (LAD)
   Severe congenital neutropenia[4]
5. Hemophagocytic disorders
   Chediak-Higashi syndrome
   Griscelli syndrome
   Hemophagocytic lymphohistiocytosis familial (HLH)[2]
   X-linked lymphoproliferative (XLP)
6. Other conditions
   CD40 deficiency[1,2,3]
   DiGeorge syndrome[1,3,4]
   Hyper-IgE syndrome[1,2,4]

---

[3] Profound T cell immunodeficiency, documented.
[4] Selected cases.

# Index

Note: Page numbers of article titles are in **boldface** type.

## A

ACK2 monoclonal antibody, for conditioning, 176
Adenosine deaminase deficiency, 211, 214, **221–236, 249–260**
    biochemical basis of, 222–223
    enzyme replacement therapy for, 225–229, 251–252
    gene therapy for, 229–231, 240–241, 252–257
    genetic factors in, 249–250
    pathogenesis of, 222–223
    stem cell transplantation for, 223–225, 250–251
Agammaglobulinemia, 243
Anemia, sickle cell, 162
Antigen presentation defects, in major histocompatibility complex class II expression
    deficiency, 174–175
Antithymocyte globulin, for stem cell transplantation, 198
ARTEMIS defects, 211, 214, 241
Ataxia-telangiectasia, 213
Autoimmune diseases
    in Wiskott-Aldrich syndrome, 181
    stem cell transplantation for, 162–163, 262

## B

B cells
    dysfunction of, in major histocompatibility complex class II expression deficiency, 175
    immunodeficiencies of, 243
Bare lymphocyte syndrome. See Major histocompatibility complex class II expression
    deficiency.
Bone marrow transplantation, versus hematopoietic stem cell transplantation, 161
Busulfan, for stem cell transplantation
    in chronic granulomatous disease, 197–198
    in major histocompatibility complex class II expression deficiency, 176

## C

Cancer, in Wiskott-Aldrich syndrome, 181
Cartilage-hair hypoplasia, 212, 214
CD3 defects, 211
CD25 deficiency, 210
CD40 ligand deficiency, 210
Chemotherapy
    for stem cell transplantation
        in chronic granulomatous disease, 197–198

Immunol Allergy Clin N Am 30 (2010) 263–268
doi:10.1016/S0889-8561(10)00034-2
0889-8561/10/$ – see front matter © 2010 Elsevier Inc. All rights reserved.

immunology.theclinics.com

# Moving?

## Make sure your subscription moves with you!

To notify us of your new address, find your **Clinics Account Number** (located on your mailing label above your name), and contact customer service at:

**Email: journalscustomerservice-usa@elsevier.com**

**800-654-2452** (subscribers in the U.S. & Canada)
**314-447-8871** (subscribers outside of the U.S. & Canada)

**Fax number: 314-447-8029**

**Elsevier Health Sciences Division**
**Subscription Customer Service**
**3251 Riverport Lane**
**Maryland Heights, MO 63043**

\*To ensure uninterrupted delivery of your subscription,
please notify us at least 4 weeks in advance of move.